Investigation into Dynamics of Ancient Egyptian Pharmacology: A Statistical Analysis of Papyrus Ebers and Cross-cultural Medical Thinking

Shingo Fukagawa

BAR International Series 2272
2011

Published in 2016 by
BAR Publishing, Oxford

BAR International Series 2272

Investigation into Dynamics of Ancient Egyptian Pharmacology: A Statistical Analysis of Papyrus Ebers and Cross-cultural Medical Thinking

ISBN 978 1 4073 0846 3

BAR Publishing is the trading name of British Archaeological Reports (Oxford) Ltd. British Archaeological Reports was first incorporated in 1974 to publish the BAR Series, International and British. In 1992 Hadrian Books Ltd became part of the BAR group. This volume was originally published by Archaeopress in conjunction with British Archaeological Reports (Oxford) Ltd / Hadrian Books Ltd, the Series principal publisher, in 2011. This present volume is published by BAR Publishing, 2016.

Printed in England

BAR
PUBLISHING

BAR titles are available from:

BAR Publishing
122 Banbury Rd, Oxford, OX2 7BP, UK
EMAIL info@barpublishing.com
PHONE +44 (0)1865 310431
FAX +44 (0)1865 316916
www.barpublishing.com

Acknowledgement

I think science-minded people often feel impelled to run statistical analysis on Egyptian medical papyri when they see the repeated occurrence of medicinal materials throughout the prescriptions recorded in the papyri. They believe they can, by such means, grasp the specific patterns and relationships that may emerge. Using a computer seems to be a very practical method, and the current advance in PC performance as well as fulfilment of applications provides us an actual opportunity to demonstrate this. However, there are obvious obstacles concerning assertions of the validity of statistical analysis as well as applications of interpretative devices to the data with the aim of bringing meaningful or new information to the study of Egyptian medicine.

Shingo Fukagawa

Kyoto

July, 2010

Contents

CD-Rom*

Data-item and arranged data-set

Title	Description	File name	Pages	Size
01) Material term and hieroglyphic writing	Identification number for each material term (TermID). Major variations of hieroglyphic spelling for the material terms in the Ebers papyrus.	01) TermHiero.pdf	17	282KB
02) Place of occurrence of material term	Prescription number where a material term occurs according to TermID.	02) TermPre.pdf	13	52KB
03) Association of source and part/product terms for detailed recognition of material	Association patterns between material terms (by TermID) for detailed recognition of material together with the prescription number where the association is made.	03) TermAssoc.pdf	16	62KB
04) Place of occurrence of material (detailed recognition)	Identification number for each combination pattern of material terms (MateID) assigned to prescription number where the material occurs.	04) MatePre.pdf	17	60KB
05) Association of materials	Association patterns of materials (MateID) together with the prescription number where the association occurs.	05) MateAssoc.pdf	230	369KB
06) Material term in the prescription	Following the prescription number, terms (by TermID) and materials (by MateID) are listed.	06) PreTermMate.pdf	70	318KB
07) Material term and frequency	Material terms (TermID) sorted by frequency (descending).	07) TermFrqSort.pdf	11	37KB
08) Material and frequency	Materials (MateID) sorted by frequency (descending).	08) MateFrqSort.pdf	15	41KB
09) Prescription, number of materials and grouping by clinical matter	Prescription number and number of materials used in each is presented together with the classification group by clinical matter of Ebbell and the *Grundriss*.	09) PreFrqMateG.pdf	16	44KB
10) Combinations of two materials and combination frequency	Combination patterns of two materials sorted by frequency (descending).	10) 2MateCombi.pdf	128	138KB
11) Combinations of three materials and combination frequency	Combination patterns of three materials sorted by frequency (descending).	11) 3MateCombi.pdf	513	509KB
12) Position of term in prescription list	Position of material term in prescription list (ascending).	12) TermPosi.pdf	67	95KB
13) Position of material in prescription list	Position of material in prescription list (ascending).	13) MatePosi.pdf	57	88KB

*Please note that the CD referred to above (and throughout the text) has now been replaced with a download available at www.barpublishing.com/additional-downloads.html

Graphics of data analysis

14) Term frequency distribution	Chart showing frequency distribution of terms in the order of prescription number.	14) TermFrqCht.pdf	9	130KB
15) Material frequency distribution	Chart showing frequency distribution of materials in the order of prescription number.	15) MateFrqCht.pdf	6	98KB
16) Dendrogram (selected analyses)	Dendrogram showing clusters of materials in groups of prescription.	16) Dendg.pdf	6	139KB
17) Correspondence analysis (selected analyses)	Graphic showing correspondence analysis for materials in groups of prescription.	17) CorrAna.pdf	68	491KB

VBA code

18) VBA codes	VBA codes used to extract combination patterns of two materials (no.10) and three materials (no.11).	18) VBA.pdf	4	58KB

Abbreviations

Bln.	=	Berlin Papyrus (3038)
Car.	=	Papyrus Carlsberg VIII
Chas.	=	Chassinate Papyrus
Cht.	=	Chester Beatty Papyri VI
Eb.	=	Ebers Papyrus
He.	=	Hearst Papyrus
Kh.	=	Kahun Papyrus
Lo.	=	London Papyrus (BM 10059)
Ram.	=	Ramesseum Papyri III, IV, V
Sm.	=	Edwin Smith Papyrus

PART 1

Fundamentals

This part sets out both the objectives of the investigation and the fundamental concepts of medicine that underpin study in the context of ancient Egyptian medicine. It begins with an illustration of the current situation of the study of Egyptian medicine (Chapter 1). This is followed by a discussion on the possibilities and effectiveness of the application of statistics as a method of future investigation in the analysis of Egyptian prescriptions. Then some key concepts derived from diverse principles of medicine known from different cultures are defined (Chapter 2). In the following section approaches are made to the Egyptian medical texts to describe their contents and introduce suggested interpretations based on the medical perspectives that have been established (Chapter 3–4).

CHAPTER 1

Statistical Approach into Ancient Egyptian Prescription

1.1 Possibilities and insights

Although less than a dozen medical papyri have come down to us from pharaonic Egypt, and certainly large numbers of Egyptian medical records have been lost, we are fortunate to have access to those texts that do remain and to have the opportunity to consult them directly and thereby gain some understanding of ancient Egyptian medicine. Following the series of discoveries of Egyptian medical papyri and their publication, various interpretative approaches have been taken by scholars over some hundred years. Although one can say that a degree of understanding of Egyptian medicine has been achieved, in fact, the opinions and interpretations vary greatly among scholars.

This is undoubtedly due in part to the difficulty in dealing with the enigmatic texts of the Egyptian medical papyri. They include many medical terms that are unfamiliar to Egyptologists since many occur only in the medical papyri, and their meaning remains unidentified or uncertain. Consequently, reading these Egyptian medical texts with their unidentifiable names of diseases or symptoms and medicinal substances is fairly often a frustrating experience. In addition, even in the case of readable texts, their ambiguity seldom allows for proper comprehension of their conceptual bases. These lexicographical and philological problems and difficulties have led to diverse interpretations, often achieved through very different approaches.

The differences in the expertise and the perspective adopted by the researchers have resulted in diverse and crucial dissensions in the interpretation of the contexts of Egyptian medicine. Quack (2003: 3–4) provides a good description of the problematic situation that confronts the students of this field:

> Die Erforschung der altägyptischen Medizin ist ein notorisch schwieriges Thema. Gerade die dabei nötige Koordinierung von Kompetenz aus den ganz verschiedenen Wissenschaftsbereichen der Medizin und der Ägyptologie ist in der Praxis schwer zu erbringen und schon gar nicht von einem Einzelnen zu leisten. Meist fehlt es dem Ägyptologen am medizinischen Detailwissen, dem Arzt dagegen am Bewußtsein für den Umgang mit zufällig erhaltenen Fragmenten, die zudem in einer toten Sprache überliefert und entsprechend problematisch zu deuten sind. Das bisherige Standardwerk zur ägyptischen Medizin, der neunbändige „Grundriß der Medizin der Alten Ägypter“, ging vorrangig von der philologischen Seite vor. Andere Forschungsrichtungen orientieren sich dagegen vornehmlich am paläopathologischen Befund. Unter diesen Bedingungen ist die Zusammenarbeit von Forschern aus beiden Bereichen prinzipiell sehr zu begrüßen … in der Praxis erweist sich leider, daß die Zusammenarbeit doch nicht die erhofften weiterführenden Erkenntnisse erbringt, sondern mithin darin stehen bleibt, bereits Bekanntes zu wiederholen. Schlimmer noch, die Kenntnisse gerade im ägyptologischen Bereich sind derart lückenhaft, daß man das vorliegende Buch nicht einmal dem zur Lektüre empfehlen kann, der nur eine handliche Orientierung über den erreichten Forschungsstand sucht.

The study of Egyptian philology is essential to properly identify Egyptian medical terms and establish a contextual perspective. The authoritative works of the *Grundriß der Medizin der Alten Ägypter* provide current definitive translations that reduce the risks of philological misinterpretation. But philology alone cannot bring about a true understanding of the medicine of the ancients, and to understand the underlying medical concepts within these texts, it is necessary to apply specialised knowledge from the field of medicine. Generally, medical specialists can apply their knowledge to paleopathology to identify diseases that existed in ancient Egypt and their command of chemotherapeutic principles can affirm the rationality of Egyptian drugs. Their assertions are usually convincing, being supported by scientific evidence. There is also a wide variety of expertise involved in the study of Egyptian medicine including that of traditional medicine, medical historians and medical anthropologists. Their understanding of Egyptian medicine provides different and important perspectives and reveals their particular methods of interpretation.

Nonetheless, it is frequently the case that the assertions among scholars show considerable differences and disagreement, and at times, the interpretations given can even be ridiculously contradictory. There seems no practical way to support a single definite and conclusive interpretation, but we should attempt to achieve a comprehensive understanding of Egyptian medicine through studying the range of understandings based on different medical perspectives. This approach should not be a problem so long as we bear in mind that these diverse interpretations are essentially hypothetical, though it is necessary to exclude unlikely interpretations that are based on mere speculative opinions. It is true, nevertheless, that the variations in interpretation often lead to confusion when an attempt to focus on the precise contexts of Egyptian medicine is made. When confronting these essential difficulties, some scholars come to the conclusion that the study of Egyptian medicine cannot form an academic discipline.

This current problematic situation in the study of Egyptian medicine seems likely to continue unless we acquire a new source of information which can provide sufficient and clearer evidence for study. Nonetheless there is room for optimism. And undoubtedly there are many aspects of research which remain unexamined in the study of this field. Quack (2003: 3) notes with regard to the possibilities for further investigation that "Einerseits sind durch bislang unpublizierte Quellen noch erhebliche zusätzliche Informationen zu erwarten. Andereseits kann man auch dem bereits bekannten Material neue Facetten abgewinnen. U.a. relevant ist die Frage der Rezeptabfolge und Textorganisation, der Bedeutung der 'magischen' Texte sowie der Decknamen für Ingredienzien. Verstärkte Untersuchungen des späten Materials werden auch die Frage nach Kontakten zur griechischen und Nachwirkungen auf die koptische Medizin in ein klareres Licht rücken."

1.2 Statistical approach as a methodology

The Egyptian medical papyri are primarily compilations of prescriptions, and the Ebers papyrus, the most important Egyptian medical text, alone employs nearly five hundred words for medicinal materials in more than eight hundred recipes. This clearly reflects the fact that the prime therapy of the ancient Egyptians resided in pharmacology. One possibility in approaching Egyptian medicine, therefore, is the investigation of particular associational patterns shown among the prescriptions recorded in the medical papyri. Treatments for ailments, ranging from internal diseases to skin disorders or traumas, are included in the prescriptions. And detailed studies have been made of the specific associations between disease and pharmacological material. Often the relevant parts of different prescriptions are listed, and sometimes quantification and calculation of the ratio of associations are provided. This approach can actually provide important criteria for the understanding of the pharmacological contexts of Egyptian prescriptions.

A notable example of such an approach is a study by Miller (1994) on an unidentified plant named *ḏaajs*. This plant appears reasonably frequently in medical papyri and also in other Egyptian writings. Miller (1994: 349) notes that "the use of *ḏaajs*-plant to expel worms in two prescriptions in the Ebers papyrus, nos. 67 and 79, provides a valuable clue to the identification of this plant." He then provides detailed notes on each instance of the use of this plant in the prescriptions by listing it along with the related disease-entities classified according to external and internal application (351–2). He notices that this plant is externally used in fumigation for schistosomiasis (Bln.59) and as an analgesic stomach cataplasm for *pnd*-worm (Eb.67) as well as a topical application for a stiff knee (Eb.605, 609), arthritis (Eb.689), refreshing the *mṯw*-vessel (Eb.95) and so on (Eb.630; He.164; Eb.522e). The cases of internal use are as an emetic, with fish and beer for stabbing rheumatic pains (*stt*) (Eb.856f), as an analgesic to reduce stomach-ache (Eb.167), to reduce abdominal swelling (*šfw.t m ẖ.t*) (Eb.587), to kill the *pnd*-worm (Eb.79) and for the treatment of an unidentified disease of the eyes (Eb.751). Further details are given of the medicinal use of its seeds (*pr.t ḏ3js*), which are employed as an internal diuretic (Eb.780) and externally for the treatment of punctures caused by an acacia thorn (Eb.732) and also for fumigation to reduce the pain of schistosomiasis (Bln.58). Another significant feature suggested is its association with another medicinal substance, notably honey. The seed appears in a salve (*gs*) mixed with honey and wax to treat polyarthritic rheumatism of the joints (*r-ʿti*) (Eb.654) and mixed with honey to ease all pains (He.94 = Eb.657 = Ram. V) as well as in the remedy claimed to be designed by the god Ra himself that also includes honey (Eb.242). Overall, Miller (1994: 352) states that the modern uses of *Peganum harmala* L. (Zygophyllaceae) correspond closely to the therapeutic contexts and preparations documented for *ḏaajs*-plant in ancient Egyptian medicine and asserts these suggest its identification.

This method of approach has, in fact, been not infrequently applied from the earliest stages in the study of Egyptian medical texts. Similar approaches to that of Millar are evident in a series of terminological studies of earlier works undertaken by Dawson (1932–35) in which he provides lists summarising the relationships of the medicinal substances with particular ailments or associated clinical matters. He also regularly notes two forms of administration of these materials (i.e. internal and external). These characteristic uses of materials are often understood from their botanical medical features.

The Egyptian prescriptions are essentially poly-pharmacological recipes that include several materials employed in a meaningful manner, composed into specific forms such as pills, a drink, fumigation, enema, suppository and ointment. Thus, it is important and relevant when studying the pharmacology of ancient Egypt based on the Egyptian prescriptions to identify the particular tendencies to associate medical substances or the relationship between the substances as well as the forms of drug composition and application. But so far little attention has been paid to the poly-pharmacological aspect of the Egyptian prescriptions, and its significance is not fully understood. Usually, it is possible to point out the active principles for one or two materials in a prescription that are mixed with a fluid substance that serves as a vehicle, like water, beer, honey and wine, without properly describing the whole value of a remedy or the functions of the other materials.

The necessity for a more systematic study of the Egyptian pharmacological aspects was asserted some three decades ago by Weeks (1976–78: 292–3):

> A major step in this direction was taken with the appearance of the fifth volume of the *Grundriss der Medizin, Die Drogennamen.* There, every drug mentioned in medical papyri was listed and briefly discussed. But, to better understand Egyptian pharmacology, we must go beyond this listing of drug names and also examine the ways in which these drugs combine with one another, the ways in which they are prepared and applied, and all the other aspects of the medical instructions that have helped Egyptian medicine achieve such renown. The kind of lexicographical study that has been applied to Egyptian pigments or to minerals is not sufficient here, because of the importance of this "environment" in which drug names occur. By "environment" we refer to all those features of a prescription that accompany a drug name and modify it: information on dosage, frequency of application, method of preparation, accompanying drugs, and another element.

The term "environment" which Weeks employs here refers primarily to the identification of particular patterns or consistencies in the Egyptian prescriptions such as the combinations of medicinal substances, their associations with diseases, composition and administration methods as well as their relationship to dosages that are frequently specified for each substance. In reality, however, such a systematic study would require considerable effort to examine the very large number of prescriptions and handle the Egyptian medical terms used in them. Weeks (1976–78: 293) notes the extraordinary requirements of such a trial study:

> Studying this environment poses a problem, however. Egyptian medical papyri refer to approximately seven hundred drugs. Four hundred of these occur in P. Ebers. These four hundred drugs are found in eight hundred of its 877 prescriptions. Each prescription contains an average of five drugs; each of these may be prepared in six different ways; administered in twelve different ways; given in six different quantities with three different frequencies to treat any of thirty major disease categories. Obviously, the number of possible combinations of these environmental attributions is large. In fact, it theoretically approaches 30,000,000,000! Of course, not all these possible combinations do, in fact, occur. And that in itself is a crucial point: there are about 300,000 combinations actually represented in P. Ebers, only about 0.1% of the theoretical limit, and these combinations are regular and recurrent.

The details of how these figures were reached are not provided, but this analysis shows that an unmanageable number of patterns would appear if all detailed specific patterns were extracted from the Ebers papyrus. Weeks (1976–78: 293) suggests using a computer as the practical method of investigation:

> Still, 300,000 is a large number, and the only practical way to identify the combinations and study their distribution is with the aid of a computer. But to write an effective computer program one must make a careful study of the data it must handle. So, before feeding this mass of information into a machine, it seemed useful to resort to old-fashioned hand sorting and see what kinds of data would result.

The purpose and intention of Weeks' article is not to present all the results of the suggested studies, instead it discusses the possibility and efficiency of performing this operation and sets out some pointers for further investigations. At the end of the article Weeks (1976–78: 297) provides several summaries of preliminary remarks on information that we could expect to gain from following these suggested courses of examination. One of the hypotheses that he notes is as follows:

> The arrangement and combination of drugs in P. Ebers suggest that drugs were systematically applied in the treatment of medical disorders by persons whose knowledge of materia medica was more sophisticated than some writers on ancient medicine have previously thought. The care shown in arranging drugs within a prescription, in noting their quantities and even, in some cases, listing and discussing alternative drugs that produce similar effects, suggest considerable experience in pharmacology. They reflect a higher degree of rational and empirical thought than we have given them credit for.

If we follow Weeks' assertion and attempt to demonstrate the examinations from which such expected results derive, we might be able to nullify the discouraging commentaries that are occasionally given in relation to the Egyptian medical papyri. These include assertions that while Egyptian medical papyri contained some common-sense remedies, many remedies were nonsense and worthless. The contents have been regarded as an admixture of absurdity by modern standards as they involve a considerable amount of magic and superstition, and by pointing out that a number of recipes can be given for the same illness, it has been thought that prescriptions were chosen *ad libitum*, and also the very multiplicity of the prescriptions is seen as a confession of their purely arbitrary character (Weinberger 1932: 58; Ranke 1941: 33).[1]

One also ought to reconsider what is regarded as the "unscientific" character of Egyptian prescriptions when pointing out the conflicting uses of some materials. The same medicinal substances are employed to function as remedies for opposing problems. The *ḏ3rt*-plant, sycamore-fig and *išd*-fruit are examples that are used both as a laxative and an antidiarrheal, and they appear in the remedies of evacuation treatment (Eb.7–43) and as a means to stop evacuation (Eb.44–8). In occasional cases the same or quite similar prescriptions are applied to very different ailments. Such features are common and rational when adopting a poly-pharmacological perspective.

It seems that, despite Weeks' encouragement for this course of investigation, the systematic full-scale study into the "environment" of the Egyptian prescriptions has yet to be undertaken. The most comprehensive statistical approach applied to the medical papyri is probably the work by Estes (1993) in which he provides percentages for the occurrences of clinical matters, the frequency of distribution of medicinal materials in the form of lists together with their suggested pharmacological property and their relative association with ailments and treatments in an appendix (136–57). He also provides some commentaries on the summaries of the statistical features. He found, for example, that honey had the highest frequency of occurrence in the Ebers papyrus with 30.3%. It was followed by the *ḏ3rt*-plant 14.6 % and frankincense 14.4% (101). The materials used primarily as solvents or diluents were noted as water 53.5%, and honey 30.3%, beer 14.5%, oil 14.5%, fat 14.3% and wine 5.2%, etc. (99). Estes (1993: 96) established that from approximately 1350 prescriptions in all the medical papyri 60% gave indications of dosage. The frequency of oral administration is stated as being 28.8% in the Ebers papyrus and 26.6% in the Hearst papyrus, topical application registers as 70.9% in the Ebers papyrus and 73.1% in the Hearst papyrus (98), which reveal a high percentage of topical application in the medical papyri.[2] The proportion of ailments when classified into nine groups of clinical matter shows 26.2% gastrointestinal tract problems followed by disorders of the skin and hair 15.7%, the limbs 13.7% and the eyes 11.2% (107).[3] As for the association of medicinal materials with clinical matters, the ratio for the occurrence of medicinal substances in relation to a further detailed classification of 16 clinical conditions was grouped into three categories of 10–20%, 20–40% and >40% (110–11). In this examination, Estes showed an association between the eye remedies and malachite of 20–40% and with Galena of >40%. Likewise, the association of gastrointestinal ailments with colocynth is 20–40%, while with the *ḏ3rt*-plant it resisters at >40%.

The statistical information provided by Estes is certainly useful for grasping the characteristic features of Egyptian prescriptions and serves as criteria in considering their possible meanings. But his statistical operations do not include all aspects of the "environment" of Egyptian prescriptions and are not fully systematic in terms of a full-scale demonstration of statistical analysis. A further difficulty is evident in that the commentaries provided are not adequately informed by an understanding of the medical principles of Egyptian prescription.

Questioning the statistical approach

There are several alternative ways to proceed with a statistical approach in order to determine and examine the "environment" of Egyptian prescriptions. One could examine the combination of materials, the position of materials in the sequence of lists, the materials' association with a specific disease and the indication of dosages. Ritner (2000: 116), however, advises caution when applying statistical operations to such studies:

> One would like a precise, statistical analysis of ancient Egyptian drugs, detailing the first introduction of each pharmaceutical and its varying frequency of application. Unfortunately, the fragmentary nature of our evidence renders the validity of such study questionable, though some broader patterns might emerge.

Ritner's cautionary remark is apposite. We possess only a fragment of the enormous body of Egyptian medical records that probably existed in ancient Egypt. Karenberg (2001: 912) notes "it has been estimated that less than 0.01% of the Egyptian medical papyri have come down to us." While this estimate lacks verification, it is very probable that our sources are equivalent to only a few pieces of an enormous jigsaw puzzle. Indeed, it is impossible to ascertain whether the medical papyri available to us are sufficiently representative of the whole range of Egyptian medicine to supply adequate results from statistical examinations. Some textual evidence in the medical papyri, in fact, reveals that they are the collection of texts/prescriptions of different temporal and geographical origins (see p. 54-5). This fact can lead to further uncertainty regarding consistency within the context of the pharmacological theory on which

[1] Erman (1894, reprinted in 1969: 360) comments "It would not however be right to deny the possibility of result to Egyptian medicine because of this admixture of absurdity. Even with the recipes described above, good cures would be possible supposing that combined with senseless but harmless ingredients they contained even one substance that was efficacious."

[2] For detail about the dosage, see p. 65-66.

[3] For a discussion about the classification of the clinical matter, see p. 74-6.

the design of the prescriptions was based. In addition, we have no clear idea about the historical process behind the compiling of the medical papyri. This raises the question of potential biases caused by the criteria which the ancient Egyptian scribes employed in their compilation process. The validity of both the statistical data derived from the medical papyri and the interpretations based on this data must, therefore, always be questioned and regarded as preliminary.

Nertheless, this does not mean that an attempt to interpret Egyptian medical papyri through a statistical approach is doomed to failure from the beginning. There is certainly room for discussion concerning this, of necessity, optimistic attempt, to evaluate and clarify the problems and possibilities of this direction as a methodology for future research. The discussions themselves can actually contribute to a meaningful understanding of the Egyptian prescriptions as well.

1.3 Statistical premise in the study of Egyptian prescription

Recognition of the medical papyri as sample bodies

The Egyptian medical papyri and their contents are fragmentary in all aspects. The difficulty in applying statistics, then, resides in the practice of regarding the medical papyri as sample bodies for analysis. Statistics, however, function as guidelines of analysis with which to extract information and make inferences from data that can be imperfect and fragmentary for many reasons. Statistics are employed in various areas of research and the business-world as a practical and effective method, particularly where it takes too much time and effort to study an entire large population or when it is practically impossible to include items which are lost.

Statistics play a significant role in dealing with partial or fragmentary data as the principle operation is to provide recognition of a "core reality" and separate that from randomness brought about by variations and errors contained in data.[4] In our case the corpus of data is comprised of prescriptions recorded in the medical papyri, and statistical data derived from them could reveal basic pharmacological trends of the prescriptions, excluding soft coating random variations (Fig. 1).

It is of crucial importance when applying statistics to consider the appropriate sampling process and potential biases that may take place in data gathering. Ideally, the sampling should be done systematically so that the sample body accurately represents the larger population. If too much data deviating from the general population is included in the gathering procedure, the statistical information and conclusion drawn from it will not accurately reflect features of the population. In this study, then, it is imperative to discuss the medical papyri in relation to the entirety of medicine in ancient Egypt, and also to discuss whether the contents of the medical papyri can be treated as representative of Egyptian pharmacological treatments in general, before moving on to demonstrating any statistical examination of Egyptian prescriptions.

Statistical data and the pharmacological perspective

Statistical operations can provide a result which reveals the trends present in the sample body. Even a failure to show a specific trend or showing strong randomness in patterns may also be forms of indication. The significance of the statistical results resides in the proper manner of interpretation, which organises the results into information capable of meaningful interpretation. Deriving statistical results and having an appropriate understanding of what the results mean are not the same thing. Here, it is crucial to have specialised knowledge of the field of study for which the interpretation of the statistical results is carried out. A medical statistical test may, for instance, indicate a strong relationship between the occurrence of cancer and a smoking habit. But this is actually merely an indication of the relationship of the two elements, and is not necessarily to be understood as stating that smoking will cause cancer, because it may also be interpreted as saying the opposite, namely that cancer can induce smoking. Therefore, with regard to the present study, we need to be sensitive to the concepts and principles of pharmacology which led to the formulation of prescriptions to be able to establish an appropriate understanding of the statistical trends derived from the Egyptian prescriptions.

[4] For a basic concept of statistics, see Siegel (1996: 2–6).

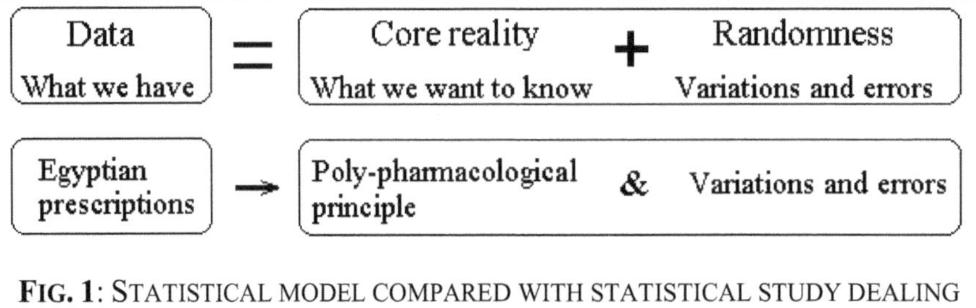

FIG. 1: STATISTICAL MODEL COMPARED WITH STATISTICAL STUDY DEALING WITH THE EGYPTIAN PRESCRIPTIONS OF MEDICAL PAPYRI.

The prime assumption which needs to be established for the interpretation of explicated statistical features with regard to Egyptian prescriptions may be viewed optimistically. Relative consistency has been attained concerning the pharmacological principles or theories on which the ancient Egyptian physicians designed their prescriptions. This is because we can assume that the Egyptians had an established medical tradition and concepts of pharmacology and that they possessed a coherent mode of prescription. In interpretation, the application of the concepts and principles of poly-pharmacology is very important as it allows us to illustrate the combinations of medicinal materials which occurred in the Egyptian prescriptions. It should be noted that this approach of engaging with and understanding Egyptian poly-pharmacological patterns is fundamentally different from the methodology commonly adopted with respect to the analysis of Egyptian pharmacology, which is a "top-down" approach where the elements "empirico-rational" or "magico-religious" properties of one material are emphasised. In contrast, a poly-pharmacological understanding of the subject is an approach from the "bottom-up," attempting to describe the association patterns of materials.

1.4 Premises and course of this work

The prime objective of this work is to consider whether the statistical analysis of prescriptions in Egyptian medical papyri can have a practical result. There are two premises that should be discussed in this regard: (1) the nature of the Egyptian medical papyri as sample bodies for analysis and (2) the perspectives of the poly-pharmacological principle which may be applied for an understanding of the pharmacological features of Egyptian prescriptions. These premises require extensive discussion that involves, as usual in this field of study, seemingly different areas of expertise.

Due to insufficient archaeological evidence for medicine in ancient Egypt and philological problems with Egyptian medical writings, we know the evidence from ancient Egypt alone cannot provide us with sufficient information to establish how fully the extant Egyptian medical papyri represent Egyptian medicine. It is therefore necessary to refer to medical writings of other cultures and by a comparative study of their nature, reaches a clearer idea of the nature of medical writings. It is useful to refer to how, in other cultures, the medicines were formulated, standardised and authorised, and also how the medical documents were complied and functioned. We may also make reference to the medical principles of other cultures in order to enhance our understanding of the Egyptian prescriptions. This study includes the cultures of ancient Greece, China and India. Of these, the Greek medical culture is particularly important, since it had a close connection with Egypt both historically and culturally (see p. 41-8). Nonetheless, medicine should be understood as an integrated aspect of culture, and it is important to note that the unique aspects of a culture can bring into being fundamental differences to other cultures. Even if we could find certain similarities on a superficial level, there may be significant differences on the conceptual level. This is a common difficulty in medical anthropology, and this is also the most difficult aspect of the current study because it involves interpretations of enigmatic Egyptian texts and includes dealing with lexicographical and philological problems as well as the anthropological difficulties of comparing different medical contexts from other cultures. For the comparison of the medical contexts, the prime sources involved are archaic types of medicine and the systematic medical theory of ancient Greek, traditional Chinese and Indian Ā*yurvedic* medicine, botanical medicine as well as the modern western chemotherapeutic medicine.

Comprehension of medical principles

Medicine is the art of healing the living body. The study of pharmacological principles alone would not lead to a proper understanding of all the underlying concepts of prescription. It actually requires comprehension of broader medical matters, especially anatomo-physiology, pathology and aetiology, because pharmacological principles and the design of drugs are directly related to them. The prescriptions compiled in the papyri should essentially be regarded as final products derived from profound consideration by physicians with broad medical knowledge concerned with the treatments of specific ailments in their patients. It would have begun with diagnostic examinations revealing symptoms and identifying the patient's pathological condition and/or related aetiological entities. Proper medicinal substances would then be selected from a broad pharmacopeia to relieve symptoms or to combat disease.

To illustrate the situation a comparison with a computer-processing model lends itself. The vast amount of data in the storage device can be compared with the broad medical knowledge of a physician. When a specific query is made, the relevant parts of the data are extracted and entered into specific formulae to be processed, just as physicians search their knowledge to understand the patient's ailments and to design a treatment. Just as a computer can provide an output which is a useful form of information, so, in the case of the physician, knowledge can produce a recipe for a drug (Fig. 2).

In order to understand Egyptian ideas of pharmacology it is necessary to deal with the contexts of the medical papyri in order to bring to bear on them all the related fields of knowledge such as anatomo-physiology, pathology and aetiology. Although the principal parts of the medical papyri are taken up by the prescriptions, fortunately for us, they do also include some important texts providing fragmentary views on these matters. Particularly important are the texts relating to diagnosis, where the manner of diagnostic examination and the symptomatic conditions as well as the pathological and aetiological entities are inferred. The medical papyri also include texts showing

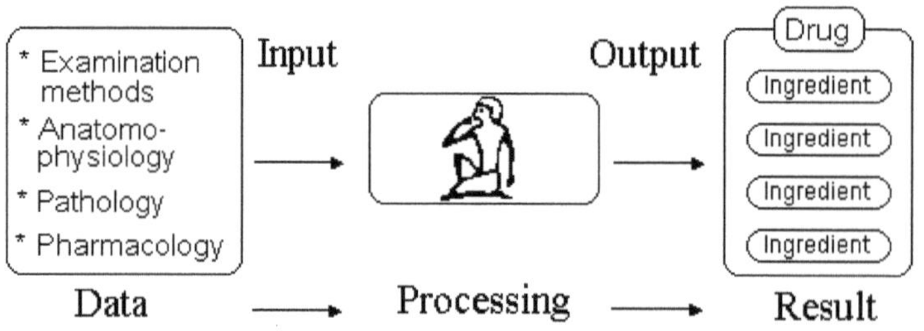

FIG. 2: PRESCRIPTION DESIGNING PROCESS COMPARED WITH COMPUTER-PROCESSING MODEL.

their views on human anatomo-physiology and their gynaecological ideas. These texts can certainly provide important clues for comprehension of the broader knowledge of medicine in ancient Egypt. But as already mentioned, these texts are enigmatic and difficult to interpret. A crucial problem is that most of such important texts are actually not explanatory but are curt descriptions of factual matters, and the interpretations of these medical contexts are problematic. So, it is useful to refer to the medicine of other cultures in this respect also.

The next step in this work is to introduce the principles of pharmacology and the concepts of disease in medicines of various kinds including primitive empirico-rational and primitive magico-religious medicine, and systematic theory of medicine as well as modern chemotherapeutic medicine (Chapter 2). These are then used as perspectives from which to describe and understand Egyptian medicine (Chapter 3–4). The following Part 2 pays special attention to the nature of medical writings in ancient Egypt. It considers their value as representative of Egyptian medicine and the extent to which they can be regarded as adequate sample bodies for statistical analysis (Chapter 5). It also explores them from the perspective of poly-pharmacological principles that are considered essential for the interpretation of the pharmacological trend of Egyptian prescriptions (Chapter 6). In Part 3 of this work, discussions on the construction of the database for the Ebers papyrus and possible statistical tests are introduced followed by some notes on technical difficulties in accommodating the contents in a database. Some preliminary statistical analyses are demonstrated and commentaries are supplied (Chapter 7).

CHAPTER 2

Medical Principles and Perspectives

2.1 Medicines for humans

People's health is vitally important not just for individuals but also for the community, to promote social life and activities. But human beings are constantly under threat of contracting diseases or acquiring injuries, and consequently the establishment of medical arts to deal with these unfortunate menaces to health has been essential. As medicine is so fundamentally important, we may be inclined to think medicine might be the oldest of any of the sciences. It might have become established prior to mathematics, astronomy or agriculture. Medicine would not have taken long to become an integral component of the larger socio-political contexts of a community. Through the course of history various forms of healing art have been devised and established, and continuing investigations into efficient therapy has led to the formulation of a "medical pluralism" where several different forms of healing exist and are practiced in a society.

One characteristic form for healing is drug therapy, in which natural and processed substances are employed and composed into a remedy. We find that the substances commonly employed can consist of those that are normally eaten as food such as celery, lettuce, meat, salt, oil, honey, beer and wine. But in a remedy such substances are quite often combined in ways that would not occur in cooking. The pharmacopeia can also include curious, uncommon and impure materials such as soot, malachite, lapis lazuli and hair, urine and even dung of animals. Other forms of medicine found in most cultures include ritual performances in which the power of incantations and protective amulets and other potentially healing manipulations and substances are employed. Dream therapy or incubation and meditations are also common methods of healing. These kinds of healing are primarily based on the belief in supernatural powers and the existence of spiritual entities. These several different forms of medicine probably co-exist in a society, and it is not uncommon for some of these to be combined in a treatment. Actually, these forms of treatment often appear to have a close relationship in their basic concept and to be inter-dependent.

The medicines of every culture are, at least superficially, similar. A quick look at prescriptions from different cultures can reveal considerable similarities in their format and the ways in which materials are used. The shamanic practices of exorcising demonical diseases and the sympathetic appeal to the divine for cure are almost universal trends. However, close studies of the medicines in each culture can reveal the presence of divergence in the role different medical principles as well as the significant differences in medicines at the conceptual and theoretical level. The principal medical concepts of different medicines are introduced in chronological order below. Interestingly enough, all these different types of medical principle can be applied for an understanding of the Egyptian medicine as it is discussed in the following section. Also, the illustration of the course of the formation of medical principles and their interaction which lead to the further development of medicine in medical history provides helpful criteria when considering the situation of Egyptian medicine.

2.2 Principles in the primitive type of medicine

Empiricism in medicine

The experience of advantageous results in successive treatments is commonly suggested as a source of medicine. Through repeated experience of intake of sycamore figs and subsequent loose stool, the laxative effect of the fig may be recognised. Or, from an accidental contact of oil with the skin, it is possible to deduce that oil can protect skin from the heat of the sun by day or enable it to withstand more easily the bitter cold by night. Usually, in the interpretation, the rational use of materials that are actually therapeutically effective is regarded as empirico-rational medicine. The use of medicinal plants such as senna, willow, cumin, cinnamon and aloe are very commonly identified with this medicine.

Sigerist (1951: 114–17) assumes that the intrinsic source of empirical medicine resides in human instincts. He mentions that man is a mammal and, like other animals, he is equipped with instincts that drive him to actions that tend to preserve the individual. Just as an animal can seek and instinctively find its food, or a newborn baby needs no instruction how to suck the mother's breast, so healthy humans seek and instinctively find animal parts, plants and minerals that are required for body sustenance. Ill humans, in a similar way, will undertake actions or instinctively find materials needed to overcome illness.

He further illustrates his views on the origins of empirical treatments with the illustration of a dog found eating herbs which could improve its condition when its stomach is upset although nobody taught it which herbs to eat. Pregnant women have been seen eating whitewash from walls because their bodies were in need of calcium. In similar ways, instincts can guide us to eat pickles when the body needs acid or to drink coffee that provides caffeine when the body needs to stimulate its slackening circulation. Similarly, spontaneous reactions such as using a hand to compress an injury would stop a haemorrhage. In the early stages one might not be aware of the therapeutic effect of such instinctive actions or of the efficacy of materials taken, but through observation, realisations could be formulated in this crudest form of medicine.

Formation of primitive medical theories

It is from the intellectual realm of the human brain that other medical principles are derived. These principles are characterised by logical conceptualisation or theorisation of ailment and therapy.

Law of similarity

One particular theorization of therapy is homeopathy, which is based on the law of *similis similibus curantur* (i.e. "likes are cured by likes").[5] This medicine uses the analogy of materials' properties including colour, form, texture, smell, name (phonetic value) and so on, and these materials are assumed to produce therapeutic effects similar to their properties which are useful for treatments. For example, red material like *geranium* or oil of *St John's wort* are used to cure disorders connected with blood or against cuts; yellow plants such as *saffron crocus* are chosen for jaundice, the white spots on the leaves of *lungwort* show that the plant is good for lung disease (Porter 1997: 38). *Anemone hepatica*, having leaves shaped like a liver, is considered to be effective for liver complaints, and *dandelion* root, with a reddish brown liver-colour, is thought to benefit the liver (Kenner 1996: 26).

Notion of supernatural entities

A peculiar feature of primitive medicine resides in the conceptualisation of the disease-entity that is theoretically handled in the treatment. For instance, a sick person should boil eggs in his own urine and bury them. As the ants ate them, the disease would also be eaten up; or similarly, to heal a swollen neck, one can draw a snake along it, put the snake in a tightly corked bottle and bury it, as the snake decays, the swelling goes (Porter 1997: 41). In these cases, the egg and the snake are used as vehicles to which the diseases are magically transferred and destroyed by being eaten up or decaying.

The notion of a supernatural entity is commonly used for the conceptualisation of disease and treatment. For instance, modern Egyptian folk medicine can explain the spiritual entity called *jinn* as a cause of a male child's disease of the throat resulting in difficulty in breathing. It claims that every child has a *jinn* sister, *ukht*, and since the *ukht* loves her brother, she tries to destroy him so that she may enjoy his love. The treatment is then cauterising the patient or scarifying his head with a razor because by doing so his *jinn* sister would take pity on him and depart from his body (Walker 1934: 46–7). The interesting point about this treatment is that the harm perpetrated against the patient is regarded as a device that serves to forcefully expel the *jinn*, the cause of disease.

Often gods or demons appear both as the causes of disease and as sources of healing. Commonly, ritual performances, magical tools such as a healing statue or wax figure, and incantations are used to combat demonic diseases with their magical power or to appeal to the sympathy of the healing gods. Mystical healing properties of materials can often be attributed to their divine associations. A typical example is the exorcising property of sanctified water. Also, many kinds of plants, precious minerals and animals that are associated with religious concepts or mythological notions are commonly found in this category of medicine.

Empirical and theoretical medicine

Both empiricism, on the one hand, and the primitive conceptualisation and theorisation of medicine on the other are based on the realization and recognition of the cause-effect relationship. But the crucial difference between them is that empirical medicine is derived from incidental or attentive observation which pays heed to interrelated facts, and empirical knowledge does not include an explanation concerning this relationship. By contrast, the theorisation of medicine aims to logically explain the mechanism of disease and treatment. In other words, the efficacy of empirical medicine is asserted merely on past experience without knowing why, although its factuality may provide conventions. Some limited reasoning ability is involved to infer the cause and behaviour of disease and to establish ways to interrupt its course. But the validity of assertions in this type of medicine may be restricted by its own conceptual framework.

On account of its practicality and rationality, empirical medicine generally possesses treatments which seem universal and that are easier to accept. But it is theoretical

[5] A similar notion known as the "doctrine of signature" is also used in the description of homeopathy.

medicine that can display greater ethnic variations due to the fact that the reasoning employed in the formation of medical theories is closely associated with specific cultural beliefs and religious concepts. It is not uncommon for the ethnicity expressed in primitive theoretical medicine to construct its practices and theories to appear bizarre, sometimes absurd and difficult for people from other cultures to understand. Nonetheless, every culture possesses this sort of primitive medicine, and despite the variations and differences in practice, the underlying fundamental concepts and principles can be identical. Thus the "weirdness" popularly attributed to the medicine of another culture is actually a form of prejudice.

A primitive type of medicine, therefore, rests on two basic medicines namely empirico-rational medicine and ethno-theoretical medicine. Ethno-theoretical medicine is more generally regarded as magico-religious medicine because the concepts used in it are mostly related to magical power or religious belief. One might regard claims that treatment by magico-religious medicine is entirely valueless and ineffective by modern standards as little more than prejudice because expectations of being cured and belief in efficacy can bring about not only emotional relief but also psychological actions that promote bodily healing action—an effect aptly known as placebo. We know the power of the placebo effect is so great that modern medical researchers have to conduct double-blinded tests to eliminate the placebo effect when the efficiency of a newly designed drug is to be tested.

Interaction of two elements

We have no substantial evidence to determine when intentional healing practice emerged in history. This could be explained by having occurred in the very remote past but it is more likely to be due to the insubstantial nature of medicine. Not infrequently paleopathological traces found in human remains reveal diseases or injuries which occurred during life, but signs of treatment that may have been taken orally or applied topically to alleviate them would have naturally disappeared in a very short period of time.

Clear evidence of intentional medical practice has only been confirmed in texts from around 4000 years ago. Egyptian medical writings recorded and preserved in several papyri and on more than 100 ostraca are certainly the earliest evidence of medicine (see p. 23-4). Also, nearly 1000 clay tablets on which medical texts were written in cuneiform have come from Mesopotamia.[6] These early records of medicines included prescriptions and incantations or other instructions for treatment of many kinds of ailment and are evidence of the early establishment of medical pluralism in the respective cultures.

Not infrequently we find that incantations are attached to prescriptions, and occasionally the magical use of wax figures is combined with drug therapy in Egyptian medical papyri.[7] The Egyptian archaeological evidence also reveals the Egyptians' use of cippus stelae[8] or other tools for healing as well as the practice of incubation cures.[9] Egyptian medicine is generally considered to be an archaic type of medicine, and the understanding of the prescriptions in the papyri is usually based on recognition of their empirico-rational (see p. 36-7) and magico-religious elements (see p. 37-8). Nevertheless it should be noted that it is probable that by the time medical practices were recorded in writing they were systematically controlled through the established bureaucratic medical institutions (see p. 56-9). Professional medical practitioners who possessed authoritative titles had already emerged at a very early stage of the dynasty (see p. 59-62). These facts require us to be aware that a separation between the mere practice of folk medicine and authoritative professional medicine took place in early Egypt even though they may have shared similar foundational medical principles.

Another relevant point is that although Egyptian medicine is sometimes used as an illustration of the beginnings of medicine in history, this view is not accurate as the actual Egyptian medical texts along with other evidence may simply indicate well-established features which reflect a long tradition of medicine. The textual studies of Egyptian medical papyri and the medical writings of other cultures indicate that they are actually compilations of earlier medicines that have been preserved through being repeatedly copied (see p. 54-5). An Egyptian text in the papyrus can even infer that that part is originated more than 1000 years before the papyrus itself (see p. 54-5). Thus it is significant to take into account the great continuity of medicine. It is possible that Egyptian medicines recorded in textual form were based on accumulated medical lores which were orally transmitted and were derived from a long medical tradition which evolved throughout a preparatory period before the invention of writing, rather than being the incidental emergence of medicine in early dynastic Egypt (see p. 9).

6 Biggs (1995: 1911–24) notes that the earliest medical prescriptions we have date from the Third Dynasty of Ur (about 2000 BC) and are written in Sumerian.

7 A fumigation treatment in the Ebers Papyrus (Eb.795), for example, uses a wax of figure of ibis, a symbolic form of god Thoth; See p. 39, 46.

8 Statue-stelae, which are also called "Horus on the crocodiles." The function of such stelae was to protect from attack by actual animals as well as supernatural beings envisaged in animal form. They were also used to cure ailments such as stings or bites (Pinch 1994: 100–3, 143–5; Nunn 1996: 107–10). Magical healing spells are often inscribed on Cippi, but Ritner (1989: 106), taking literacy rate into account, notes that the efficacy of the spells was rather transferred to a more practical medium by pouring water over the stelae or by immersing them in a bowl of water, and then the water was drunk by the patient in hope of cure. The basin for the collection of water can be seen at the feet of the healing statue of Djedhor (Cairo Museum, jdE 46341) (Nunn 1996: 112).

9 The practice of sleeping in a temple in the hope of having a dream in which a deity would indicate a cure. The inscription of the stela of Qen-her-khepeshef (19th Dy) may be an early account of this practice, but otherwise it is not proven before the Late Period (Nunn 1996: 110–11).

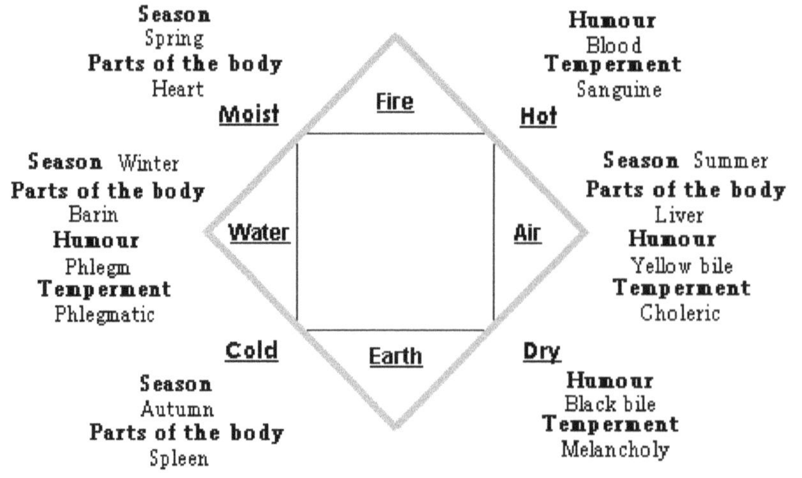

FIG. 3: THE GREEK COSMOLOGICAL MODEL SHOWING ITS ASSOCIATION WITH MEDICINE (BASED ON CHEVALLIER 2000: 33).

The historical continuity of medicine can result in certain difficulties in ascertaining the pure elements of empirico-rational and magico-religious medicine. In the course of transmission, the initially empirically-derived medical knowledge would have become anecdotal knowledge shared in a community. Variations and modifications may have been added to an original magico-religious theory to enhance and ensure its efficiency by followers of that practice. And it is highly probable that the empirical and theoretical elements were tightly interwoven in such a way that the empirically derived knowledge of medicinal material was provided with a sound explanation through its association with magical and religious concepts, or a material of magico-religious property might reveal actual effectiveness by chance, thereby enhancing the convention of its theory. There may have been even more complicated processes during the development of medical knowledge where several principles interacted and were combined, and where further innovations in treatment based on the older medicine were promoted. The occurrence of variations and modifications and the creation of new treatments together with the concomitant persistence of older medicines could lead to a multitude of medical treatments in a culture.

2.3 Systematic theory of medicine

Interesting coincidences have occurred in the development of similar systematic theories of medicine in Greece, China and India in the period from *ca* 500–200 BC, although little is known about the origins and early stages of the art in each of these cultures. Medicine was recorded in classic texts known as Hippocratic corpus in Greece, *huang di nei jing* (黄帝内経 "*Yellow Emperor's Inner Canon of Medicine*") in China (Hongtu 1999: 1–2), and *Caraka Samhitā* and *Suśruta Samhitā* that formed the bases of Āyurvedic medicine in India (Keswani 1967: 76–8; Basham 1976: 18–21). In general, it is considered that the systematic medical theory of these three civilizations is relatively independent, but the considerable similarities and shared features have led to the assumption about possible historical links between these cultures. Opinions vary greatly. Some scholars do not exclude the possibility of foreign stimulus, especially of Ionian Greek philosophy influencing Chinese medicine; others see an Indian influence on China via Buddhism, while some assume an Indian influence on the Greeks. One also finds assertions of influence in the opposite direction.[10]

The emergence of systematic medical theory brought a phase of innovation to medical history. The principle feature of this medicine is found in a theory based on a holistic and systematic model of a cosmological philosophy where symbolic cosmological elements are bound and governed by universal law. Brief descriptions of the characteristic theory of each medicine are provided below.

Ancient Greek medicine

Greek natural philosophy consists mainly of the four cosmic elements *fire*, *air*, *earth* and *water* together with the four primary qualities, *hot*, *cold*, *dry* and *moist*; these

[10] There are many arguments concerning the possible origin of the systematic theory. For example, Unschuld (1985: 54) states "The origin of this innovative development, beginning with the late Chou, are not sufficiently documented in ancient Chinese sources to allow for any definitive identification. The possibility of a foreign stimulus cannot be excluded. It is commonly accepted that the rise of philosophy in the Ionian sphere, that is, the step from *mythos* to *logos*, dates back to influences originating from some other cultural center, farther to the east. Ionian Greek philosophers took up what they learned from outside, developed it further, and gave it its characteristic Greek appearance. They were not ashamed of having assimilated outside thoughts; on the contrary, they were proud to have refined what was brought to them in a rudimentary state ... A philosophical impulse may have spread from one unknown source somewhere between Greece and China ..."; Lesile (1976: 2–3) notes Indian influence on Greek medicine indicated by the fact that several Hippocratic authors recommend medications that they attributed to India, and he also assumes its influence on Chinese medicine via the diffusion of Buddhism to China, and he comments "yet Chinese medicine had no discernible effect on the development of Āyurveda."

are arranged in a stylised model of a symmetric grid that represents the basic structure of the universe (Fig. 3).

All sorts of natures in the universe are then attributed to the four properties recognised by their association to the nature of the four cosmic elements, such as the four seasons of the year, the four temperaments (sanguine, choleric, melancholy and phlegmatic) or more specifically the four ages of man (infancy, youth, adulthood and old age). In this systematic theory all the natural phenomena are involved in serving as the components of the universe, and all phenomena of the universe are explained through the versatile systematic associations of these components. The striking aspect of this theory is the holistic integrity with all natural phenomena included in the theoretical model, and all natures systematically related and in correspondence according to the cosmological law that maintains a state of equilibrium in the universe (see p. 67-9).

Medicine is one of the components contained in this systematic theory, and it is understood in much the same way as the other sciences based on this cosmology. The Four-Humoral Theory of the Hippocratic school of Cos is commonly used to show the systematic medical theory of Greek medicine. In the Hippocratic corpus (460–377 BC), the four cardinal humours—blood, phlegm, yellow bile (or choler) and black bile (or melancholy)—are identified as essential constituents of the body, and its texts repeatedly emphasise the importance of the harmonious balance between the humours for health. Just as natural disasters or destructive phenomena are understood to happen due to the disequilibrium of cosmic elements, so the loss of balance from excesses or deficiencies in one or more humours would result in diseases.

There could be many causes of the humoral imbalance. One example that reveals the holistic integrity of the humoral pathology with regard to natural phenomena is the seasonal causes. In the Four-Humoral Theory, two qualities are attributed to each humour. Blood was considered a mixture of hot and moist natures, phlegm of cold and moist, yellow bile of hot and dry, and black bile of cold and dry. The nature of these humours correlates with the natures of four seasons. Phlegm increase during winter because, being cold and moist, it is akin to the chilly and rainy weather of winter; and colds, bronchitis and pneumonia are then more prevalent. When spring comes the blood increases in quantity, and diseases follow from a plethora of blood, increasing spring fever outbreaks, dysentery and nose-bleeds. By summer the weather is hotter and drier, the yellow bile increases, and so disease resulting from yellow bile multiplies, such as severe fevers. In the cooler autumnal weather the yellow bile declines but in turn black bile increases bringing its symptomatic diseases (Porter 1997: 60).

The role of medicine, then, was to restore the balance of humours. The holistic aspect of systematic theory leads to diverse approaches which give attention to food, exercise, sleep, repletion, evacuation, emotional and sexual habits. In pharmacological treatment, the restoration of the equilibrium of humours is also sought and a prime property based on four cosmic qualities is attributed to medicinal materials. In treatment, the material of contrary quality is applied so as to counterbalance the existing excess or deficiency of humours. We can occasionally find qualities ascribed to materials in the Greek texts, as we read, for instance, advice to "apply warming substance" as noted in the Hippocratic corpus (*Places in Man* 346–8) that include cow's dung, bull's gall, myrrh, alum (Potter 1995: 99).

Chinese medicine

The earliest textual evidence indicating a formation of Chinese systematic medical theory dates to around 200 BC.[11] This medicine is based on the Chinese cosmological notions of *yin-yang*[12] and five phases (*wu xing*).[13] The *yin-yang* theory is a dualistic cosmology where the universe is recognised as consisting of manipulations of binary opposites (Fig. 4).

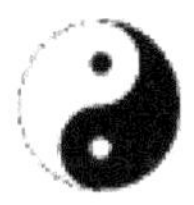

FIG. 4: THE SYMBOL OF THE DUAL COSMOLOGY OF YIN AND YANG, ILLUSTRATING THEIR MUTUALLY DEPENDENT NATURE.

This cosmology involves pairs of opposites such as *heaven* and *earth*, *sun* and *moon*, *night* and *day*, *winter* and *summer*, *male* and *female*, *up* and *down*, *inside* and *outside*, and *movement* and *stasis*, etc., and such extreme opposites are theoretically associated as being mutually complementary in that they depend on and counterbalance each other, thereby creating the equilibrium of the cosmos.[14] In medicine, diseases are classified according to the nature of *yin* or *yang*; interior, vacuity and cold diseases, for instance, are *yin*, and the exterior, repletion and heat diseases are *yang* (Wiseman 1995: 2). *Yin* and *yang* natures are also ascribed to pharmacological materials, and as a surfeit of *yin* or *yang* is a cause of diseases, hot diseases are cured by cold materials and cold by hot materials.

[11] Unschuld (1985: 54–5) notes it as the second half of the last millennium BC.

[12] *Yin* and *yang* are the words which literary mean "shadow" and "light."

[13] The translation of the term *wu xing* as "five phases" is to reflect the dynamic notion inherent in the Chinese term *xing* which literally means "to proceed," and the translation as five elements is avoided in general; Yanchi (1998: 3) states "Through the theories of vital essence and qi, yin and yang, and the five elements as the theoretical methods and holistic concept, The Yellow Emperor's Internal Classic explains the law of life, and the unity of the body with the natural world."

[14] For a detailed description of *yin-yang* theory, see Yanchi (1998: 21–35).

The Five-Phases Theory is a cosmological paradigm of five constituents that are symbolically expressed as *fire*, *earth*, *metal*, *water* and *wood*. Similar to the Greek model of the four cosmic elements, Chinese cosmology is used to define and explain all natures through the illustration of the interaction of the five phases attributed holistically to all phenomenal matters including seasons, colour, flavour and so on (Tables 1 and 2).

Wood	Nourishing and flourishing
Fire	Hot and flaming upwards
Earth	Nourishing and cultivating
Metal	Astringing and reforming
Water	Moisturizing and flowing down

TABLE 1: NATURES OF THE FIVE PHASES IN CHINESE COSMOLOGY.

Phases / Phenomena	***Wood***	***Fire***	***Earth***	***Metal***	***Water***
Season	Spring	Summer	Long summer	Autumn	Winter
Weather	Wind	Heat	Dampness	Dryness	Cold
Direction	East	South	Centre	West	North
Development	Birth	Growth	Maturity	Withdrawal	Dormancy
Colour	Green-blue	Red	Yellow	White	Black
Tastes	Sour	Bitter	Sweet	Acrid	Salty

TABLE 2: FIVE-PHASE CATEGORIZATION OF PHENOMENA (BASED ON WISEMAN 1995: 16).

There is considerable resemblance between the Greek and Chinese theories in that all phenomenal matters are holistically integrated into one model. An example from Chinese theory shows how the constituents of the cosmos can be structurally and mechanically associated and interact with each other.

In Chinese cosmology, four theoretical cycles exist that express the associations among cosmic constituents; *engendering*, *being engendered*, *restraining*, and *being restrained* (Fig. 5). *Engendering* denotes the principle whereby each of the phases produces, nurtures and benefits another phase. *Restraining* refers to the principle by which a phase constrains another phase.

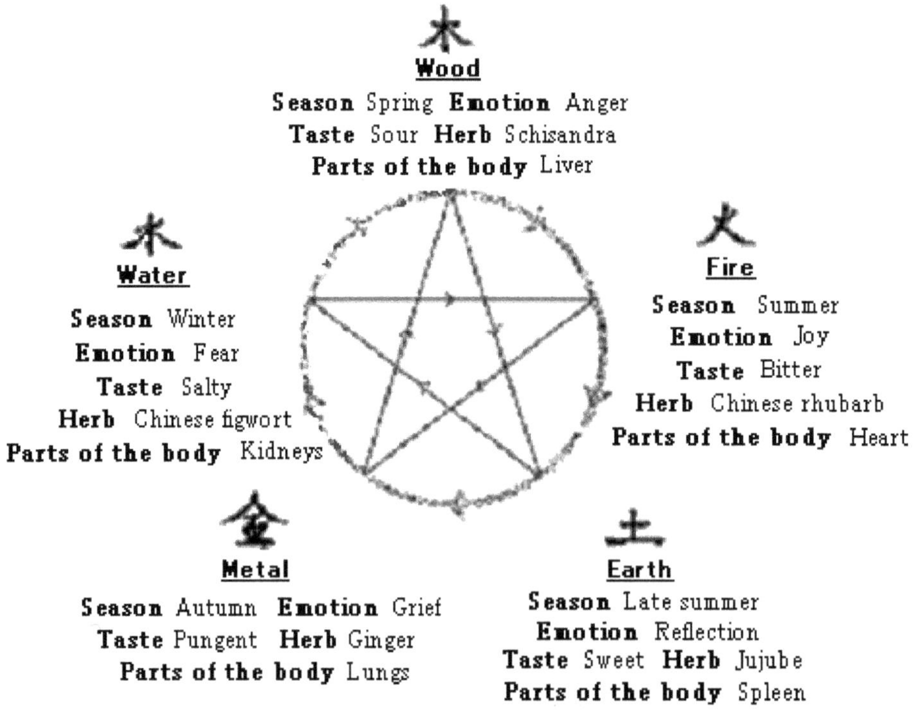

FIG. 5: CHINESE COSMOLOGICAL MODEL REPRESENTING THE FIVE PHASES AND THE ENGENDERING AND RESTRAINING CYCLES (BASED ON CHEVALLIER 2000: 41).

Phases / Human nature	*Wood*	*Fire*	*Earth*	*Metal*	*Water*
Viscus	Liver	Heart	Spleen	Lung	Kidney
Bowel	Gall bladder	Small intestine	Stomach	Large intestine	Bladder
Sense organ	Eye	Tongue	Mouth	Nose	Ears
Tissue	Tendon	Vessel	Muscle	Skin/hair	Bone
Emotion	Anger	Joy	Pensiveness	Grief	Fear
Voice	Shout	Laugh	Sing	Cry	Groan

TABLE 3: FIVE-PHASE CATEGORIZATION OF HUMAN NATURE (BASED ON WISEMAN 1995: 16; YANCHI 1998: 43).

The arrangements and relationships of the constituents in the correlation cycles are explained in Chinese theory as follows:

- **Engendering cycle:**

Wood → Fire → Earth → Metal → Water → Wood
(Wood brings forth fire; fire produces ashes, that is, earth; earth can produce metal; when heated, metals produce steam, that is water)

- **Restraining cycle:**

Wood → Earth → Water → Fire → Metal → Wood
(Wood will be cut down by a metal tool; the metal will be broken by fire; the fire is extinguished by water; the water will be exhausted by the earth; the earth will be loosened by wood) [15]

The two aspects of *generation* and *restriction* in this theory are especially significant because these create an indispensable correspondence system that formulates the mutual balance of the cosmic constituents. *Wood*, for example, generates fire, and on the other hand, it restricts *earth*; while *earth*, in turn, generates *metal* and restricts *water*; and the phase restricting *wood* is *metal*, and the one that generates *wood* is *water*. Therefore, the phases in the theory of systematic correspondence oppose each other and at the same time cooperate with each other, and this enables the establishment and maintenance of the equilibrium of the universe.[16]

In Chinese systematic theory the *yin-yang* and five phases are inseparable principles, and the successful combination of these theories reveals a great depth of thought and tradition. In medicine, the *yin-yang* theory is applied to the human body where, for example, the abdomen is *yin* and the back as *yang*, and the five viscera are *yin* and the six bowels are *yang*.[17] In the theory of the five phases internal organs and other aspects of human nature are associated with the natures of the five phases (Table 3).

The anatomo-physiological concepts are established and described in ways similar to the systematic theory of cosmology. The liver, for example, is recognised as being *wood* in nature, and it relies on the kidney *water* for nourishment. The liver stores the blood in order to support the heart. The heart, being a heating agent, also transports its nutrients to replenish the lung. The lung provides a clearing and descending property due to its metallic nature and it then assists the flow of water to the kidneys. The generating and restraining correlations among the internal organs are the following:

- **Engendering:**

Liver → Heart → Spleen → Lung → Kidney → Liver

- **Restraining:**

Liver → Spleen → Kidney → Heart → Lung → Liver

Usually the engendering and restraining associations can maintain mutual relationships and maintain a harmonious balance among the bodily five phases that brings health. But when one of the five phases becomes excessive or insufficient for some reason, pathological conditions emerge. For instance, the overflowing of kidney *water* can be restrained by spleen *earth* via the liver because *wood* can loosen *earth* which in turn enables it to subdue the excessive moistening function of the kidney. When the situation becomes out of control and malfunctions of the mutual relationship occur, the overflowing of kidney *water* first brings harm to the liver.[18] And the damaged function of the liver in turn can lead further damages to other organs that will result in the development of disease.

Just as in Greek medicine, Chinese medicine regards many sorts of internal and environmental agents such as seasonal, and climatic factors as possible causes for diseases from

15 For clarity, the description of association of phases in the restraining cycle is given in reverse order.

16 For a detailed description of the Five-Phases theory, see Yanchi (1998: 40–61).

17 The five viscera are the heart, liver, lung, kidney and spleen; the six bowels are the stomach, large and small intestines, gallbladder and bladder, and triple burner.

18 For a detailed description of interaction among viscera based on the cycles of five phases, see Wiseman (1996: 8–12).

Doshas / Phenomena	Vata	Pitta	Kapha
Season	Rainly	Fall	Spring
Day and night	Afternoon	Midday/Midnight	Before noon
Age	Old Age	Adult age	Yong age

TABLE 4: CLASSIFICATION OF THE TIME FACTORS ACCORDING TO *TRIDOSHAS* (BASED ON WARRIER 1997: 50).

disequilibrium. The treatments are also designed based on the theory of systematic correspondence, so that diseases of abnormal sufficiency or deficiency are treated through manipulation of the engendering and restraining correlation of the related phases. This is typically achieved by the application of drugs which possess one or more of the natures of the five phases. An example that shows the holism of Chinese pharmacological treatments is the use of the property of the test of a material in association with the five phases, so that the therapeutic action of drugs with bitter taste are defined to act on the heart; sour drugs act on the liver; sweet drugs act on the spleen, and so on.[19]

Āyurvedic medicine

Indian Āyurvedic medicine also has many features comparable to those of the systematic theories in Greek and Chinese medicine. The five cosmological constitutions (*mahābhūta*) structuring the universe are *ether* (*ākāśa*), *air* (*vāyu*), *fire* (*agni*), *water* (*āpaḥ*) and *earth* (*pr thivī*) (Obeyeskere 1976: 201). The natures of these constituents are then applied to the understanding of anatomo-physiology so that *ether* is resident in the cavities of mouth, abdomen, digestive tract, thorax and lung. *Air* is manifested in the movements of the muscles, pulsations of the heart, expansion and contraction of the lungs, the workings of the digestive tract and the nervous system. *Fire* is manifested in the digestive system, metabolism, body temperature, vision and intelligence. *Water* is present in the digestive juices, salivary glands, mucous membranes, blood and cytoplasm. *Earth* exists in the nail, skin and hair as well as in the elements that hold the body together: bone, cartilage, muscles and tendons (Chevallier 2000: 37).

The Three-Humours Theory in the medicine of Āyurveda is somewhat similar to the Greek humoral theory, but its uniqueness is expressed through its fundamental concept of the *Tridoshas* (i.e. "three forces"). The *tridoshas* are three essential forces that are formed through the combinations of the five cosmic constituents. From *ether* and *air*, the air principle *vata* is created; *fire* and *water* yield the fire principle *pitta*; *earth* and *water* produce the water principle *kapha*. Each *dosha* has its own unique nature, but together they establish the mutual interrelation and equilibrium of the universe (Chevallier 2000: 37). Just as in Greek and Chinese systematic theory, Āyurveda exhibits the holistic integration of natures in its theory (Table 4). In the medical doctrine, the three humours namely *wind*, *bile* and *phlegm* are correlated with the nature of the *tridoshas* and described as essential forces that govern all biological, anatomo-physiological, and psychological functions of the body.[20] It emphasises, as in other systematic medical theories, the importance of the balanced condition of *wind*, *bile* and *phlegm* for normal health, and how any deviations result in illness,[21] and pharmacological considerations based on the notion of *tridoshas* exhibit considerable similarity to the pharmacology of Greek and Chinese medicine.[22]

The essence and principles of systematic medical theory

The descriptions of the Greek, Chinese and Āyurvedic medicines presented above are brief and simplified, and they neglect both chronological and geographical variations for each of these long standing medical traditions. But for our purpose it is sufficient to grasp the fundamental concepts and principles of the systematic medical theory. The essential components underlying the systematic theory based on cosmology are the primary cosmic elements and the law of the universe that sets the systematic and mechanical correspondences of the constituents, neutralising the excess or deficiency of a constituent and producing mutual harmony in the universe.

Another important aspect of systematic theory is the notion of macrocosm and microcosm. It is this notion that leads to the incorporation of different natures and the establishment of a dynamic relationship among the natures where things are governed by the same law. Often this notion is applied to the socio-political structure describing the law-governing arrangements and functions of a harmonious society (see p. 69-70). The human body, being a microcosm, is therefore governed by same cosmic law. Thus, in medicine, the anatomo-physiology, pathology

[19] Hongtu (1999: 41–7) introduces the medicinal property of Chinese materia medica based on theories in The Yellow Emperor's Canon on Internal Medicine; For a detailed description of Chinese theory on drug properties, see Xingdon (1998: 7–19).

[20] *Caraka* (i.9.4) reads "Discord … is disease, concord … is health," and *Caraka* (iv.5) expresses the view man is the microcosm of the universe; and just as the universe was subject to the law of cause and effect, and functioned according to regular rhythm, so was the case with man (Basham 1976: 22).

[21] For more details about Āyurvedic medical theory, see Basham (1976) and Obeyeskere (1976).

[22] Chevallier (2000: 38–9) provides a brief description about attribute of medicinal properties; For a basic concept of Indian pharmacology, see Meulenbeld (1987).

and pharmacology are understood as being based on cosmological principles.

The simplest form of recognition of pathological conditions in the *yin-yang* theory is the recognition of a diseased nature according to the prime quality of *hot* and *cold*. But Chinese medicine commonly classifies diseases into four categories: *hot*, *warm*, *cool*, and *cold*. These qualities are based on the assumption of qualities that "*yang* in *yang*" is to be *hot*, "*yin* in *yang*" is to be *warm*, "*yang* in *yin*" is to be *cool* and "*yin* in *yin*" is to be *cold*. The *hot* and *warm* or the *cold* and *cool* differ in potency. In pharmacological treatment, the therapeutic effects of medicinal substances are also classified according to the *yin-yang* theory. The *yin* substances are used to treat heat syndromes, and conversely the *hot* and *warm* of *yang* are used against the cold syndromes. This is somewhat similar to the Greek systematic theory of medicine where clinical conditions and pharmacological substances are aligned with the four qualities of *hot*, *cold*, *dry* and *moist*, and the *hot* diseases are cured by a *cold* remedy, *moist* by *dry* and vice versa (see p. 67-9). This pharmacological treatment can be aptly regarded as allopathy, which operates on the principle of *contraria contraries curantur* (i.e. "contrary treatment cures contrary symptom"). Although it appears fairly simple in principle, its actual practice in pharmacology can involve very complicated considerations and operations (see p. 68 n. 207). One reason for this complexity, in the systematic theory of medicine in general, is that several qualities can be attributed to one single medicinal material in varying degrees, so for instance, musk was hot and dry in the second degree, and cucumber is cold and moist in the second degree. In addition, multiple assumptions derived from the other kinds of pharmacological properties like tests, and other qualities assigned through holistic association with natural phenomena are common. The numerous exceptional cases established in each doctrine of medicine reveal the depth of medical thought.

Systematic medical theory is commonly evaluated as being "rational." This rationality is emphasised not because of the established "effectiveness" of treatment—as in the case of the empirico-rational medicine—but because of the implicit theoretical rationality which contrasts with the non-rational magico-religious theory. One significant aspect of the systematic theory is its systematic and holistic understanding of the cause-effect relationship among all phenomena within the structured relationship of cosmic constituents and established cosmic law. The recognition of cause and effect in primitive magic stands basically on a single-linear relationship of the two elements, and in many cases the event brought about through the magical relationship is a particular independent phenomenon in itself and does not include any associations with other kinds of phenomenal matters. An understanding of relationship in primitive magic is often based on arbitrary reasoning. Systematic theory, by contrast, forms a geometric structure of correspondences of phenomenal elements and expresses a coherent order of cause and effect, and many diverse phenomenal matters are holistically associated in the theory.

Systematic theory is also often regarded as "scientific" in terms of its freedom from religious notions. In primitive cosmological philosophy, the cosmic forces and cosmic law are described as involving the participation of divinities who govern the universe, and all phenomena are understood as being manipulations by the gods. Such understandings are often illustrated in religious and mythological texts. Thus, in primitive medicine, medical theories include demonical pathology or treatments by a mystical divine power based on magical and religious concepts. Sometimes medical historians, pointing out these primitive empiricism and irrational magico-religious beliefs, regarded primitive medicine as "pre-rational" medicine, and in order to discern the significant innovative step leading, in medical theory, to the formation of a systematic medical theory—commonly associated with the Greek contribution—primitive types of medicines, including ancient Egyptian medicine, are sometimes referred to as "pre-Greek" medicine.[23]

Nevertheless, it should be noted that earlier traditions of medicine or religion persisted even though systematic theory could have eliminated the recognition of divine influence in its theory. Even Hippocratic medicine was institutionally centred on the religious cult of Asklepios, the patron deity of the physician; and in the writings of the Hippocratic corpus we can find invocations to Apollo and the oath to Asklepios (see p. 59). In fact, medicine in Greece, China and India could include demonical diseases, homeopathic healing and other forms of magical treatment that continued being practiced even after the formation of the systematic medical theory. Not infrequently we actually find incantations or instructions for ritual performance in the Greek, Chinese and Indian medical texts. Much evidence has been found for the Greek practice of incubation. The great durability of older medical traditions and their co-existence with newly formulated systematic medicine in a culture serves to enrich medicine and develop broad medical pluralism.

Cultural elements in the systematic medicines

There are certainly considerable similarities between the Greek, Chinese and Āyurvedic medical theories. Just how similar their medical writings are would become immediately apparent if we simply replace the key terms in the text from one culture with the notions from another—

[23] Longrigg classifies medicines in ancient Egypt and Mesopotamia into "Pre-rational and irratianal medicine" mentioning, "In both of these ancient societies diseases were held to be manifestations of the anger of the gods. The physician's role was to appease the god and drive out the demon possessing the sick person's body" (1998: 5), and the achievement of "rationality" is attributed to the Greeks "The ancient Greeks were the first to evolve rational and theoretical systems of medicine free from magical and religious elements and based upon natural causes" (1998: 18).

Greek with Chinese, Greek with Indian, or Chinese with Indian. The writings would still make sense, which leads to the idea that they might either all have a single origin, or that the sporadic occurrences of similar theories in separate cultures may be mere coincidence.

Due to the lack of evidence concerning the early formation of systematic medicine in all these cultures, it is difficult to draw conclusions. We should, nonetheless, consider the possibilities of cultural association and interaction in which the gradual exchange and influence of knowledge among cultures occurred and through which the formation of similar systematic theories was achieved.

It should be noticed, however, that there are also significant differences in the medicines of these three cultures. There are certainly identical terms, like "air" or "heat", or similar explanatory texts of the theory of medicine among their medical writings, but their meaning may have quite different significance. Bile or phlegm, for example, can be found in the Greek theory of humours and in Āyurvedic medicine, but its meaning can have a different significance. The notion of bodily vital force, that also plays an important role in the medicines of the three cultures, is called *pneuma* in Greek, *qi* in Chinese and *prana* in Āyurveda.[24] There are similarities among these, but misconceptions may occur when the significance of their differences are not understood. The translation of these term into the western concept of "energy," for instance, can lead to obvious misunderstandings for someone who has no access to ancient or traditional culture. Thus, there are always medical anthropological difficulties and problems occurring when we deal with the similarities and differences in medical texts and in their contexts within different cultures. We should be aware that in some cases, specific medical terms should not be translated and must be understood by the original terms, particularly when the terms express specific cultural notions, even if they are translatable.

Modification of medical ideas through transmission

A medicine, as mentioned above, is essentially integrated within the context of a culture, and the diversity of medicines in cultures reflects indigenous ethnicities. This means any comparative study of medicines must of necessity include considerations of aspects and concepts particular to the respective culture. Also, the aspect of modification and variation must be considered which is repeatedly applied to the medicine in the course of transmission of medicine.

The systematic theories of Greek, Chinese and Indian medicine became the prevailing and dominant mainstream medicine of each civilization, and it was not long before they also became highly influential in neighbouring countries as well as in the medicines of later periods. The Greek Four-Humour Theory was largely accepted by physicians of the Roman Empire (100 BC to 400 AD). Galen (129–?199 AD) is an eminent Roman physician who followed Greek medicine and wrote numerous medical books in which the clear influence of Greek medicine, particularly of the Hippocratic corpus, is shown.[25] He is also known for his development and expansion of medical ideas although the essential elements of medicine remained relatively static. With the collapse of the Roman Empire attention to examples of medical history shifts to the East. Greek medicine was transmitted by Arabs who referred the medicine as *yunānī-tibb* ("Ionian medicine") in Arabic. Many classical Greek medical texts and also Galen's works were translated into Arabic. The authoritative Arabic medical work *Al-Qanun fi'l-tibb* (القانون فى الطب "*Canon of medicine*") by the well-known Arabic physician Ibn Sina (Avicenna; 980–1037 AD) was in large part derived from Galenic medicine.[26] During the Byzantine Empire the *yunānī-tibb* supported the Golden Age of Islamic medicine. Later in the Middle Ages, the classic Greek texts and Galen's texts were translated back into Latin from Greek and Arabic, and Greek medicine was then diligently applied to European medicine. Even in the 17th century, students in university medical schools were given academic training in principles of Greek humoral medicine. These historical courses are evidence of the great continuity of medicine over 1500 years and the strong line of transmission of medical literature beyond country and language.

Traditional Chinese medicine still plays an important role in medicine in China, and its influence is particularly strong in medical institutions in Korea and Japan. Traditional Korean medicine *Hanui* and Japanese *Kanpoh* were formed on the basis of Chinese medicine (Porter 1997: 148). Chinese medicine was first brought to Japan in the 5th century AD by Buddhist monks from Korea. In the following centuries Japanese students were sent to China to learn Chinese culture and medicine. However Japanese physicians started to assert their own cultural identity, and *Kanpoh* developed its own characteristic traits, emphasising the Japanese ideals of simplicity and naturalness.[27]

Āyurvedic medicine was most influential in Southeast Asia, and it is still playing a major role. Āyurveda was known in the Mediterranean region long before the translation of the Greco-Roman medical texts into Arabic. Several Hippocratic authors recommended medications that they attributed to India. But later, the Greek influence came into Asia in the form of *yunānī-tibb* from the Islamic tradition, and in some places like Sri Lanka the practice

[24] The concept of "vital force" found in these medicines is not included in the discussion in this work, rather the emphasis is on the role of the notion of cosmic law in their medicine, which has certain parallel in Egyptian religion and cosmology.

[25] On Galen and his works, see Edelstein (1970: 454–5) and Rhodes (1985: 19–23).

[26] On Ibn Sina, see Rhodes (1985: 25–6).

[27] About the Chinese influence and the development of *kanpoh*, see Otsuka (1976).

of both *yunānī-tibb* and Āyurveda can be found, and some degree of interaction between them can be recognised there. But no translation of the Hippocratic corpus has so far been found in India, although some scholars assume influences from Galenic works in the Āyurvedic medicine of a later period (Meulenbeld 1987: 2).

Many studies on medical history and medical anthropology have revealed interfusion and interaction of different medical cultures through which complex development and modification of medical ideas were achieved in each culture.[28] Unschuld (1985: 55) writes "the travel of ideas is different from the travel of merchandise. The latter can be handed on, from one region to the next, by different means of transportation, without itself undergoing any change. Ideas must be transmitted by the head, and, of necessity, will undergo change."

2.4 The chemotherapeutic principle of western conventional medicine

Western conventional medicine, regarded as a truly scientific medicine, emerged around the 17th and 18th century in Europe. The noticeable features of this medicine are the identification of germs, virus and bacteria that are ultimately responsible for causing infectious diseases, and the identification and understanding of pharmacological chemicals and their therapeutic actions. The fundamental scientific aspect of western conventional medicine resides in its manners of investigation by which research is founded on high standards of objective reproducible evidence in laboratories (evidence-based medicine). Enormous advances have been made with the application of microscopic observations and other forms of sophisticated implementations, and remarkable progress has been made in understanding the causes and nature of diseases as well as human anatomy and physiology. Pharmacological research has become focused on chemotherapeutic principles where isolation and purification of chemicals are carried out, and their therapeutic effects are evaluated in deliberate clinical tests (see p. 64–5). The major source of chemicals are secondary metabolites of plants. In contrast to primary metabolites that are ubiquitous chemicals in plants for normal growth, the secondary metabolites are chemical compounds developed to defend against herbivores and pathogens or to survive in interspecies competition. The wealth of chemicals in plants is explained by the fact that plants are rooted to one spot and cannot fight or flee from predators. They are, therefore, especially dependent upon chemical defence.[29] Thus, many chemicals that are extracted from plants are actually poisonous, but when they are used for therapeutic purposes, they can kill infectious bacteria or fungi and stimulate internal organs.

The chemotherapeutic principle and empirico-rational elements

It is through this chemotherapeutic principle of western conventional medicine that we can recognise the empirico-rational elements of the ancient or traditional medicines. In a study the confirmation of empirico-rational elements is made through recognition of the active chemical components contained in the plants or substances of other kinds, and by noticing the proper uses of the chemicals in the treatment against the proper ailment. An interesting correspondence between western conventional medicine and ancient, traditional medicine is their high reliance on plants as a pharmacological source.

Although the chemotherapeutic principle is an important criterion for the recognition of empirical elements in the study of ancient and traditional medicines, we tend to evaluate the medicinal materials of older medicine as "non-scientific" when their pharmacological applications do not parallel those of conventional medicine. This is actually an attitude of the modern scientific ego. The rise of western conventional medicine is only recent, and despite its progress and the accumulation of medical knowledge occurring at an ever-increasing rate, our pharmacological knowledge of chemotherapeutic principles is still in its infancy. The crucial problem is that our knowledge of the total effect produced from complex chemical interactions resulting from combinations of a number of different chemical components contained in a plant is quite limited, and the evaluation of the actual therapeutic effectiveness as shown by a whole plant is assessed only insufficiently (see p. 64–7).

The chemotherapeutic principle and traditional medical theory

Further dramatic advances in western conventional medicine were made during the 20th century. The technical advances in molecular biology, metabolic engineering, biochemical genomics, chemical analysis and other forms of clinical examinations are remarkable, and the achievement of detailed knowledge of the human body, diseases and chemotherapy have opened up a new phrase in the history of medicine. This is often referred to as a therapeutic revolution. It has been highly valued and adopted throughout the world.

---

28 Ghalioungui (1968: 105) states "it is quite erroneous to think of ancient cultures as discrete cases isolated by forbidding 'terrae incognitae.' The conditions that permitted the centrifugal spread of man since his emergence were equally permissive at all epochs and in all directions. Our ancestors were as inveterate travellers as we are today. Travel was only slower."

29 Bennett *et al.* (1994: 617–18) notes that "The term 'secondary metabolite' is rather unsatisfactory, as it covers somewhat indiscriminately a very wide variety of unrelated compounds and implies a secondary, unimportant role for them. In the past such secondary metabolites have been viewed as waste products resulting from 'mistakes' of primary metabolism, and therefore of little importance to plant metabolism and growth. It has become clear that such views are largely inaccurate and misguided, and that many secondary products are key components of active and potent defence mechanisms—part of the age-long 'chemical warfare' fought between plants and their pests and pathogens."

Nevertheless, it is only in the last 50 years that western medicine has become the norm, and estimations have been made that about 75% of people in the world do not have access to western medicine, and many rely on medical traditions that evolved during antiquity (Raskin *et al.* 2002: 522). Traditional medicines are particularly active in Asian countries. Traditional Chinese and Āyurvedic medicine are largely practiced and continue to flourish today in China and India. In Sri Lanka the *yunānī-tibb* still plays a major role; and we should attend to the fact that these traditional medicines are seldom regarded as being non-beneficial, irrational or inferior to western medicine. In recent times, more medical scholars are seriously studying the medicine and pharmacological materials of older traditions. The practitioners of traditional medicine in China and India in particular are conducting extensive research into their materia medica, with the intention of re-evaluating and proving the efficacy of their treatments from a modern scientific point of view.[30] Also, due to the recent increase in popularity of traditional herbal medicine in European countries and America, the study of medicinal plants is receiving much attention there.

In the drug industry, the importance of investigation into traditional medicinal substances is also recognised, and many plant chemicals have been identified, isolated and purified, but the emphasis has gradually shifted from extracting compounds from plants to making their analogues synthetically from simpler organic reagents (see p. 64-5). But plants are still a prime source for the discovery of new active components. About 250,000 plant species contain a much greater diversity of chemical compounds than a chemical library (Raskin 2002: 524). The investigation of plant chemicals is a highly competitive field, and plants found in all sorts of environments such as the deep sea, rain forest, higher mountains and hot springs, along with organisms ranging from bacteria and fungi to plants are now being studied. But some researchers are paying particular attention to plants known from traditional medicine as they think these are more likely to provide the historically proven effect of chemical compounds contained in traditional medicinal plants (see p. 65).

A number of studies of chemical compounds extracted from plants have been reported, and not infrequently the pharmacological effect of some chemical compound is confirmed in clinical tests, providing proof of the pharmacological efficiency of a plant. But usually the practitioners of traditional medicine ascertain that they obtain superior results with whole extracts rather than with isolated compounds from the same plant. This fact is considered to be due to a synergistic effect resulting from the interaction of chemical components contained in a plant. This synergistic effect is still mysterious to us, and we must consider the complex situation by which several medicinal materials are employed, as in the case of traditional prescriptions that commonly employ more than two materials (see p. 66-7).

Another important point is that although the chemotherapeutic principle can—to a certain degree—provide confirmation of the effectiveness and rationality of a traditional medicine, its description of rationality does not refer to its theoretical side (see p. 21 n. 35). In fact, in traditional medicines, medicinal substances are given their pharmacological values as defined by the cosmology based in systematic theory. It is not uncommon, however, that while the use of medicinal materials from traditional medicine is often thoroughly rational, its theory remains irrational. Nonetheless, we may understand this feature to be a result of empirically derived rational knowledge that is accommodated and integrated into the theoretical framework of medicine. It is, therefore, important to be aware of the complex relationship between the empirico-rational elements and theoretical aspects of medicine as well as the difficult situation in studying and understanding the many aspects of a medicine. One may notice, for instance, that a judicious use of herbal or mineral substances in a traditional medicine can modulate the immune response to infectious diseases, but this finding of rationality does not necessarily mean the practice of empiricism without theory. But at the same time it need not be immediately suggestive of the existence of concepts of immunology in the medical theory.

Dynamic medical pluralism and medical interfusion

Starting from simple empirical practices or shamanic ritual healing, many forms and variations of medicines have been formulated in the course of medical history. As described above, older practices may have persisted though with some modifications, even after newer forms of medicine were established, and every culture necessarily possesses multiple forms of medicine. This situation has not changed. Magic has maintained a powerful sway in medicine throughout history and is by no means extinct today, even among civilised nations. Many simple herbal medicines remain in the form of folk medicine. The emphasis on homeopathy appears from time to time since its origin in ancient time and its revival by the well-known physician Paracelsus (1493–1541) in the Renaissance[31] and the German physician Samuel Hahnemann (1755–1843). Hahnemann's homeopathic principle is slightly different from the homeopathy that is described above. He asserts that a substance that causes particular symptoms in a healthy person cures a sick person with the same symptoms.[32] Modern homeopathy is largely based on

[30] An interesting example is the experiment by Jagtab *et al.* (2004) where a polyherbal āyurvedic formulation for inflammatory bowel disease is scientifically evaluated and its efficacy is confirmed.

[31] On Paracelsus and his works on medicine, see Clendening (1960: 95–105).

[32] Hahnemann first provided evidence from experiences to support his medicine. He knew that mercury was commonly used to treat syphilis and noted a similarity between syphilis symptoms and those of mercury poisoning. Consequently he investigated many materials to confirm this sort of relationship (Shelton 2004: 15).

his teachings and is popularly practiced particularly in Germany. The practices of aromatherapy that use aromatic essential oil extracts from plants for healing are also popular in western counties.[33] The continued practice of traditional medicine found in Asia and also in some other countries in conjunction with modern medicine has already been mentioned above.

It is the cosmopolitan culture of modern societies and the vast increase of interest in complementary and alternative medicine (CAM) that has led to a dynamic modern medical pluralism.[34] It is particularly in the past 20 years, through the active and extensive exchange of cultures among countries, that the increasing adoption and popularity of other cultures' medical practices has been reported. CAM comprises a diverse set of therapeutic practices that are considered outside the norm of western conventional medicine. One may include Chinese acupuncture, Indian yoga and reflexology developed in England.

Also, as is always the case, the interaction and interfusion of the different systems of medicine is occurring at the present time. One form of current interfusion of medicine is known as "syncretic medicine," which combines the best of the synthetic drugs of modern medicine and of the medicinal substances from traditional medicine. Some countries in Europe allow physicians to prescribe botanical drugs together with synthetic drugs (see p. 64 n. 196), and drugs compounded from synthetic drugs and *kanpoh* materials are popularly consumed in Japan.[35]

2.5 Medicine, science and religion

Occasionally rigorous study of traditional medicine has revealed some traditional therapies to be ineffective or sometimes even harmful. In such cases they are evaluated as "non-scientific" or "irrational" treatments; or one may regard them as "magical" or "religious" because the notion of "irrational science" is often replaced by that of "magic" or "religion." The concept of what is "scientific" or "rational" would be the most difficult to define. The quality of being "scientific" and "rational" is commonly ascribed to Greek medicine by medical historians, but it would appear to the "unscientific" and "irrational" from the modern scientific point of view. Thus recognition of what is "scientific" and "non-scientific" can vary depending on the perspective applied.

The notions of the "scientific" and "non-scientific" or "religious" are essentially opposing perspectives. It is because we tend to see science and religion as separate and contradictory paradigms. In antiquity, however, there was no line distinguishing between science and religion. Religion was a vehicle of science, and science was a device to support religion, and we should be aware that the essential purpose of both science and religion is to identify truth and explain reality (see p. 50-2).

We know ancient people were keen observers of natural phenomena that occurred around them. In occasional situations they must have been able to find a mysterious coincidence or regularity in phenomena. For instance, the ancients may have noticed the coincidence of celestial movements and seasonal cycles or the regularity between celestial phenomena and the annual flooding of a river. The ability to establish such factual realities must have relied on scientific observation. It was this type of knowledge that could lead to the understanding of the world. But for the ancients, all natural phenomena are the manifestation of divine forces. Thus the investigation into the true aspect of natural phenomena is to interpret a mysterious divine force, and becoming aware of the regularity of the universe is to know the divine law that governs the universe. While modern scientists apply their command of physics, chemistry or mathematics to understand the natural phenomena observed, the ancients applied logical conceptualisation with the notion of supernatural power to understand them. We can see that the recognition of the factual event may remain the same both in the modern and the ancient approach. A superstitious teaching may give a warning not to cut too many trees in a forest because it can bring the anger of a god of the forest and result in a huge flood or the drying up of the river as a punishment, while modern scientists may emphasise the significance of the ability of the trees to keep the water in the forest. Therefore the descriptions of the universe or the behaviours of divinities in the ancient mythological texts may appear "religious" to us but would have been "scientific" for them. This is the integrity of science and religion in antiquity, and medicine is a scientific component of the religious dimension in antiquity, and we may think of other branches of science such as astronomy, mathematics, geometry and even music as well as socio-politics and economics, that are now regarded as separate disciplines, but were all closely associated with religion in antiquity. So it should be emphasised that although the concepts of "scientific" and "magico-religious" could serve as indications of "scientific" and "non-scientific" elements in a medicine, this recognition would not be appropriate when we think of medical theory and the principles of ancient medicine as

[33] The prevailing notion of aromatherapy is a treatment through the sense of smell, but the plant essence is actually administered in a variety of ways internally and externally including vaporizations and suppository (Kenner 1996: 15).

[34] The terms "complementary" and "alternative" are generally used interchangeably. Bryant *et al.* (2003: 55) make a distinction between them— in "complementary" medicines, some scientific documentation exists, and the practice may be integrated in mainstream health-care practice, whereas "alternative" medicine refers to practices that are either scientifically unfounded or lacking in support data. They note complementary therapies include massage, relaxation, herbal therapy, acupuncture and hypnosis, and other therapies such as homeopathy are classified under the alternative label.

[35] Otsuka (1976: 336–7) points out that in the study of the pharmacological substance of *Kanpoh*, the most characteristic features of its theory and principle have been laid aside for they can hardly be proven by the available methods of natural science, even though they can be empirically recognized. He quotes words from an old article by a Japanese pharmacologist Inoko (1891): "Chinese and Japanese drugs have not been studied by foreign scientists. Perhaps they contain pharmacologically active substances. But if some effective substances are discovered, they must be used according to the principle of Western medicine" (1976: 335).

understood in antiquity, and this premise is very significant when we consider the medical knowledge and practice in ancient Egypt (see p. 48-52).

The different medical principles introduced in this chapter are all important perspectives for a study of the Egyptian medicine, for an application of each individual principle to the corresponding context in Egyptian medicine can contribute towards a different approach and understanding of Egyptian medicine; thus the following chapters deal with the interpretation of Egyptian medicine based on these medical principles.

CHAPTER 3

Reading and Understanding Egyptian Medical Texts

3.1 Egyptian medical texts as a source of information

Returning to Egyptology, in this section we consider the context of ancient Egyptian medicine. Due to the scarcity of substantial evidence concerning ancient medicine, this study of Egyptian medicine relies heavily on the Egyptian medical texts that are recorded on papyri and ostraca. The principal medical papyri are Kahun, Ramesseum, Edwin Smith, Ebers, Hearst, London, Carlsberg, Berlin and Chester Beatty papyri (Table 5).[36] These papyri can be roughly characterised by their contents which are classified according to the clinical matters. In general they consist of compilations of prescriptions that treat a range of ailments, and this feature of the medical papyri may indicate that the essence of Egyptian medicine resided in pharmacological treatment.

Most of the prescriptions have quite a simple textual format. An indication of the symptom or the ailment to be treated is given in the title followed by a brief list of the names of materials, sometimes with specifications of dosage, and short instructions for composition and application are noted at the end. In many cases, the title is abbreviated simply stating "another" or "another remedy." This may mean that the remedy is an alternative treatment for the ailment noted above. The composition and application methods may be similarly abbreviated by the use of the expression "likewise." As an example, for a stomach ailment, a decoction of cumin, goose-fat and milk is recommended (Eb.5), while other remedies have an exotic appearance, such as a drink prepared from the

[36] Leitz (1999) has published fragments of magical and medical papyri of the New Kingdom held in the British Museum (BM EA 9997+ 10309, 10042, 10059, 10085+10105 and 10902) (see p. 54 n. 141); Westendorf (1999: 4–79) provides precise information of many medical papyri and ostraca.

Title	Approximate date	Contents
Kahun	1820 BC	gynaecological
Ramesseum III, IV, V	1700 BC	gynaecological
Edwin Smith	1550 BC	surgical
Ebers	1500 BC	general medical
Hearst	1450 BC	general medical
London (BM10059)	1300 BC	mainly magical
Carlsberg VIII	1300 BC	gynaecological
Berlin	1200 BC	general medical
Chester Beatty VI	1200 BC	rectal disease
Ashmolean Museum	300 BC	general medical
Brooklyn snake	300 BC	snake bite
London and Leiden	250 AD	general medical and magical
Crocodilopolis	150 AD	general medical

TABLE 5: CHIEF EGYPTIAN MEDICAL PAPYRI (BASED ON NUNN (1996: 25) WITH ADDITION OF THE PAPYRUS ASHMOLEAN MUSEUM*).

*On Papyrus Ashmolean Museum, see Quack (1991).

testicles of a black ass (Eb.756) and a black lizard which is designed to cure baldness (Eb.469). Such indications of an ailment and instructions on the composition of a remedy, however, do not reveal the important conceptual part of the treatment, and although we may frequently be able to point out empirico-rational elements or magico-religious components in the materials of a prescription, such simple recognition of elements is obviously insufficient to describe the essentials of Egyptian pharmacology. This is because such an approach fails to take cognisance of the fact that the course of treatment is usually closely related to or based on ideas of the human body and the concepts concerning the causes and behaviour of diseases. The pharmacology is, in other words, a logical designing of treatment based on anatomo-physiology and pathology together with knowledge of the medicinal properties of materials (see p. 7-8). A remedy is intended to fix the abnormalities which have occurred inside the body or combat the disease-entities. When we attempt to understand Egyptian pharmacology, it is therefore necessary to comprehend at least the fundamental ideas of Egyptian anatomo-physiology and pathology.

A major difficulty is that unlike the Greek medical texts that explain their medical ideas, or Chinese and Āyurvedic medicine where teachings are still preserved and transmitted to present practitioners, no text that systematically explicates the conceptual part of anatomo-physiology and pathology is included in the Egyptian papyri (see p. 24-7). There are, however, some important texts in the medical papyri that provide us with fragmentary views and ideas of Egyptian anatomo-physiology and pathology (see p. 27-36). These provide significant clues on which we can develop an interpretation of medicine in ancient Egypt. For some hundred years, dedicated studies have been undertaken on these texts. But as previously mentioned, reading and understanding Egyptian medical texts is quite problematic, due to the fact that only a very limited portion of medical terms have been securely identified and many terms still remain uncertain, and in many cases scholars have presented alternative interpretations. Sometimes these different interpretations of a text are the result of a different understanding of its grammatical structure.[37]

Making a sound translation alone would hardly be sufficient to elucidate the medical contexts. For instance translation alone, without context, does not supply us with sufficient information to fully understand a text describing the difficult pathological situation of a woman who is required to be treated by a fumigation remedy applied "into her vagina (*iwf*)" in order "to cause a woman's womb to go to its place (*h3j*)" (Eb.795) (see p. 38, 46-7).[38] This example illustrates that the true difficulty appears when we need to interpret the texts within their medical context, and doing so can only be achieved through the application of the medical perspectives of other cultures; yet the medical anthropological difficulties and the risk of having misconceptions resulting from cultural bias and preconceptions must always be taken into consideration.

Before moving into the study of the contents of the medical papyri, I would like to draw attention to a possible case of misconception derived from a preconception. The profession *swnw*[39] is commonly translated as physician. But from archaeological evidence we know that priests, especially of Sekhmet and Serqet, and magicians were also practitioners of medicine in ancient Egypt (see p.27 n.50). This fact is well illustrated in a text from the medical papyri which states "if any *swnw*, and *wꜥb*-priest of Sekhmet or any magician places his hands or his finger upon (a patient's) head ..." (Eb.854a; Sm.1).[40] The physician, priest and magician are clearly distinct qualifications, but we do not know if there were any significant differences in their methods of treatment. It may be a misconception to conclude that the *swnw* practiced rational prescriptions and the priests and magicians were relying on magical healing.[41] When we consider the integrity of science and religion in antiquity, it should not come as a surprise if a *swnw* employed a ritual healing or if a priest prescribed a rational remedy.[42]

3.2 Contents of and clues in the medical papyri

Before discussing the methods employed in interpreting the contents of medical papyri, the important key terms of the Egyptian anatomo-physiology, pathology and pharmacology are introduced which are essential to the understanding of Egyptian medicine.

Egyptian terms of anatomo-physiology

A good number of anatomical terms are found inside and outside the medical papyri. The Egyptian language possessed a rich array of anatomical terms for which more than two hundred anatomical parts have been identified. The list includes ordinary internal organs such as the heart,

[37] The authoritative works of H. Grapow, H. von Deines and W. Westendorf, *Grundriss der Medizin der alten Ägypter*, although about 30–50 years old, still form a fundamental and reliable basis for the textual study on the Egyptian medical papyri.

[38] In this work, the translation of papyrus Ebers is chiefly based on that of Ghalioungui (1987) and Ebbell (1937). Some parts are my own translation based on Wreszinski's (1913) Hieroglyphic transcription.

[39] Jonchkheere and Westendorf prefer the transliteration *sinw*, which is closer to the Coptic word for doctor ⲥⲁⲉⲓⲛ or ⲥⲏⲓⲛⲓ (Erman 1951: 427) and gives some indication of the likely pronunciation (Ghalioungui 1983: 1; Nunn 1996: 115); Miller (1991) follows this transliteration.

[40] In this work, the translation of Edwin Smith papyrus is mainly based on Breasted's (1930) translation.

[41] It was in fact the physicians who had double or even triple qualifications, as in the case of *Wenen-nefer* who bore the titles of priest of Sekhmet and inspector of physicians; *Nedjemqu* who was the chief of the priests of Sekhmet and chief of physicians, and *ḥeryshefnekht* who was the chief of the magicians, high priest of Sekhmet and the Pharaoh's physician (Ghalioungui 1973: 14).

[42] In the context of this work, I use the term "physician" to mean the medical practitioners including *swnw*, priest and magician in this work.

lung, stomach, liver, spleen and bladder; but many other terms exist which represent very specific anatomical parts. There is not always agreement on their precise meaning, and many still remain unclear and uncertain.[43] Nunn (1996: 49–51) supports the identification of *gmꜥ* (Sm.18) as the zygomatic part of the temporal bone, *tpꜣw* (Sm.7) as flax cerebri and *ntnt* (Sm.6) as the brain membrane. The significant point to be drawn from this is that the Egyptians were able to differentiate and name a great many organs and organic structures, and these specific terms were understood when reading the text, though such terms might have been be recognised only by physicians. This observation is an indication of the depth of Egyptian anatomy.[44]

There are important paragraphs entitled "Treatise of the heart" included in the Ebers (Eb.854–6), Edwin Smith (Sm.1) and Berlin papyri (Bln.163) that provide glimpses of Egyptian physiology. The term *mṯw* is used to describe the interconnected structure of physiology. The *mṯw* is a difficult term to translate accurately for it seems it can represent any sort of tubular vessels inside the body, and it is usually translated simply as "vessels." In the texts, the heart is described as the central organ, and the *mṯw* that initially spread from the heart into the organs and body parts could interconnect the organs and function as the transportation vessels for blood, air and various other fluid substances. It states, for example, that "there are 4 *mṯw* in his nostril, 2 give mucus and 2 give blood (i.e. epistaxis)" (Eb.854b), "there are 2 *mṯw* to his testicle, (and) it is they which give semen" (Eb.854i), and also "there are 2 *mṯw* to the bladder, (and) it is they which give urine" (Eb.854n). The meaning of these texts is relatively easy to grasp, and we can understand the proper relationship between the organs and the substances mentioned in the texts. But some texts are difficult to interpret as in the case of 4 *mṯw* that carry water and air to the liver (Eb.854l) and to the lung and spleen (Eb.854m). One text mentions that all *mṯw* are united to the anus (Eb.854h).[45]

Symptoms and diseases in the Egyptian texts

Various kinds of symptomatic conditions and ailments are mentioned in the medical papyri. These are sometimes expressed in ordinary words but more often by specific terms that are quite unfamiliar to us. Many important clues to the identification of diseases and the Egyptian's concepts of disease come from the diagnostic texts. The Edwin Smith papyrus regularly provides a diagnostic section with a description of the condition of trauma before the instructions for treatment are given, but most prescription texts in other papyri assume that the diagnosis has already been made, and the symptoms and the ailments are simply noted in the title (see p. 32). However, there are some parts where diagnostic descriptions of the ailments are presented. The diagnostic texts have a stock expression that begins with "if you examine a man with" followed by the description of the symptoms as though a master was giving an instruction to his pupil. Often the study of a diagnostic text also reveals the diagnostic methods that the Egyptian physicians employed in their diagnosis (see p. 26). Less commonly we find other kinds of texts that provide a brief explanatory gloss which is useful in making interpretations (see p. 30, 34, 36).

Descriptions of symptoms and diseases

Clinical consultation, in which a physician reveals a symptomatic condition through conversation with his patient, seems to have been a method of diagnosis in ancient Egypt. A diagnostic text of the Edwin Smith papyrus records an injury which "is painful when he hears speech" (Sm.21). Patients' complaints to the physician about their illness include such statements as "it is painful when something enters into it (stomach)" (Eb.206), "he is too oppressed to eat" (Eb.188), and "all his limbs are heavy for him" (Eb.189).

The physician seems to have interrogated his patient. An instruction is given: "you should ask her (patient) 'what do you smell?' if she says to you 'I smell burnt meat ...' " (Kh.2). Sometimes directions are given by the physician to elicit the patient's responses, e.g. the physician says "look at your two shoulders (i.e. shake the head right and left)" and then he finds "should his doing so be painful (even though) his neck turns around a little for him" (Sm.19). Similarly, the physician commands "extend now your two legs (and) contract them both (again)" and here we can see the patient's contracting his/her legs immediately after extending them because of pain (Sm.48).

In some cases it appears that the patient's condition was so serious he became unconscious and the physician was unable to get a response. Loss of consciousness due to severe injuries was recorded in the Edwin Smith papyrus: "if you call to him (and) he is speechless (and) he cannot speak" (Sm.22), and "if you ask him concerning his malady and he speaks not to you" (Sm.20). Texts that can be taken to express lack of consciousness due to illness are found in the Ebers papyrus, e.g. "his mind goes away" (Eb.198); another refers to the "perishing of the mind" (Eb.855u).

The physician's eyes played an important role in the observation of abnormalities in the appearance of the patients. In the Edwin Smith papyrus the descriptions

[43] For the Egyptian anatomical terminology, see Grapow (1954), Lefebvre (1952) and Walker (1996).

[44] Evidence of anatomical research is not found from pharaonic Egypt, except the record of Manetho which refers to an anatomical study by king Athothis (see p. 57); The practice of mummification in ancient Egypt is often assumed to be a source of anatomical knowledge, but Westendorf (1992: 46) mentions not much of anatomical knowledge could have been derived from the practice of mummification that "Aber selbst der Paraschist, der den Leib aufschneiden mußte, hat gewiß aus religiöser Scheu den Leicham über das für die Mumifizierung notwendige Maß nicht beschädigt, um dem Toten einen (möglichst) unversehrten Leib für die erhoffte Wiederauferstehung zu lassen."

[45] For a detailed discussion on the organs and substances associated with the function of *mṯw*, see Nunn (1996: 44–9) and Westendorf (1999: 119–22).

of conditions of injuries are frequently graphic, and we can easily visualize the situation. A severe head injury is described by the words "a swelling protruding on the outside of that split, while he discharges blood from his nostril and from his one ear having that split" (Sm.21). In other cases abnormal symptoms caused by traumas are apparent on the face: "his eye is askew because of it (a smash in the skull)" (Sm.8) and "both his eyebrows are drawn, while his face is as if he wept" (Sm.7). The abnormal skin symptom of an internal disease is described as "on his back like the trouble of one who has been stung (by an insect?)" (Eb.200). Changes in colour mainly of the skin and also the eyes were observed in a patient who, for example, "has changed and has turned deathly pale" (Eb.198), or shows "ruddiness of face" (Sm.7) and "his eye on the side of him having that injury is bloodshot" (Sm.19). A curious skin symptom can be "on his shoulder, his arms, on his sacral region and his thighs that there is colour" (Eb.877b). Also, a large swelling is mentioned as being "motley-coloured" (Eb.874). Abnormal behaviour due to ailments is observed: "his belly is narrow and he is miserable to go like a man suffering from burning in the anus" (Eb.188).

The application of a physician's hands in the diagnosis is also indicated. The records of the medical papyri describe the abnormalities sensed by a physician including a wound that "something disturbing therein (wound) under your finger" (Sm.4), "it (swelling) goes and comes under your fingers, and it is divided by your hand when it is fixed" (Eb.867), "it (enlarged gland) is as if there are cloths in it, it is soft under your fingers" (Eb.857). The patient's reaction when being touched is also recorded, "you should press the manubrium of his sternum with your finger, he shudders exceedingly" (Sm.40). The symptoms from internal diseases recognised by the physician's hand are "his body all through is shivering when your fingers are applied to him" (Eb.193) and an abnormal belly condition is described as "it (stomach with a resistance) goes and comes under your finger like oil in a leather bag" (Eb.199). The examination of the temperature of body parts was also an important diagnosis as we see in the following texts: "it (a tumour) is very hot therein when your hand touches him" (Sm.39) and "you find them (tumours) very cool" (Sm.45). A strange symptom of an internal ailment can be that "you find the two sides of his belly: the right one warm and the left one cool" (Eb.188).

We can also find the use of the sense of smell in diagnosis. The text of the Edwin Smith papyrus mentions "the odour (of a suppurated wound) of the chest of his head (i.e. "crown") is like urine of sheep" (Sm.7) and "a finger or a toe that is ill, fluid (i.e. "pus") goes around them, (and) their smell is bad" (Eb.617). The Ebers papyrus notes an ill person's breath is "like a latrine" (Eb.190).[46]

The texts of medical papyri therefore reveal that Egyptian diagnosis was achieved chiefly through a clinical consultation and ocular, olfactory and tactile observation. These observational methods may appear as crude, but actually represent very basic diagnostic methods still employed today. The abnormal smell of a patient is still recognized as an important diagnostic sign. For instance, a stinking smell from the phlegm of a patient can suggest the possibility of suppuration in the bronchial tube. Sigerist (1951: 328) notices the resemblance in the diagnosis by pointing to the Egyptian text that describes an enlarged gland like a kind of fruit (*ỉrtjw ḫsd*) (Eb.858), and he mentions "we also compare tumours with fruits all the time and describe one as having the size of an orange, another as being like a cantaloupe."[47]

Names of symptoms and diseases

The Egyptian medical papyri include many terms that appear to represent specific symptoms or diseases, though many remain unclear and uncertain for us. They are understood through contextual interpretation, or the nature of the symptom or disease is roughly understood from the determinatives that are attached to the terms, e.g. the terms with a determinative of fire 𓊮 (Gardiner sign-list: Q 7) may be related to a heat symptom or a disease such as a fever or an inflammation.

One group of terms that appears to be related to ailments are those with the determinative of a snake 𓆙 (Gardiner sign-list: I 14) including *ḥft* (e.g. Eb.5), *pnd* (e.g. Eb.82), *ḥsbt* (e.g. Eb.102), *bṯtw* (e.g. Eb.205), *sꜣ* (e.g. Eb.617), *sp* (e.g. Eb.617), *fnt* (e.g. Bln.20; He.196; RaIII.B, 3). These terms are commonly understood as representing specific species of parasitic worm. The infectious disease caused by parasitic worms is still common in present-day Egypt, and it must have been common in ancient Egypt, as we have several instances of evidence of worm infection revealed through the pathological examinations of Egyptian mummies. Ruffer (1921: 17), for instance, found a large number of calcified ova of *Schistosoma haematuobium bilhazia* in the kidney of two mummies of the 12th Dynasty, and Tapp (1979) discovered the larval form of *Strongyloides*-worms in the intestinal wall of a mummy of the 25th Dynasty. The adult parasitic worms of many species are around 1–2cm in length[48] and often visible to the naked eye wriggling under the skin, around the eyes and nose, and occasionally in stools. So, the ancient Egyptians may have had opportunities to observe the worms. Since parasitic worms such as the roundworm, threadworm, hookworm, pinworm and segments of tapeworms had a very distinctive appearance, it is possible that Egyptians recognised the species and gave them individual names. Ebbell (1937) provides some

[46] Ebbell (1937: 48) translates "his breath-sides is like a latrine-cave," but Ghalioungui (1973: 77) and Pahor (1992: 680) interpret that the patient's breath was compared to the smell of a latrine.

[47] Sigerist's commentary is based on Ebbell's (1937: 121) identification of *ỉrtjw ḫsd* as a fruit of *calotropis procera*. But Grapow (1962: 669) translates *ḫsd* as "Geschwulst" and Ghalioungui (1987: 234) translates the words as "(*ỉrtjw*) of *ḫsd*-swelling," which would not allow Sigerist's comparison.

[48] Nunn (1996: 70) mentions that species such as female *guinea*-worm can attain a length of upto a meter.

identifications, e.g. for the *ḫft* as a roundworm and the *pnd* as a tapeworm. But such identifications are often questioned due to lack of a firm basis. But Sigerist (1951: 332–3) follows Ebbell's identification, stating that the *ḫft*-worm, as it is designated by the same word as "snake" could indicate it was a roundworm, and the *pnd*-worm is probably a tapeworm. Nunn (1996: 72) suggests that these terms might be considered as the names of internal disease caused by worms.

In the incantation texts contained in the verso of the Edwin Smith papyrus the word *ṯ3w* ("wind" or "air") is employed in association with a disease. The incantations are said to be designed against the "wind of *i3dt* (i.e. the pest) of the year" (Sm.verso.XVIII.1–XX.11). The texts can sometimes take abbreviated forms like against "the pest of the year" and simply "this year" or in other parts alternatively "evil wind" (Sm.verso.XVII.8) or "plague-bearing wind" (Sm.verso.XVII.11). The "wind" here is considered to be a poetical expression for annual epidemic disease (Breasted 1930: 473). It may be possible that the Egyptians associated air with disease through the attentive observation of the aerial infection of epidemics. And actually, this association is commonly made in medicines of various cultures.

While such an association may be based on the mere observation of nature and behaviour of the annual epidemic, it would certainly not include a knowledge of bacterial or viral infection. The ancient Egyptians seem to have attributed the epidemic wind to divine causes. One incantation mentions that it is to expel "the plague-bearing wind, the demons of disease, the malignant spirits, messengers of Sekhmet" (Sm.verso.XVIII.11–12), and the spell to be recited is "I am Horus who passes by the diseased one of Sekhmet. Horus, Horus, healthy despite Sekhmet" (Sm.verso.XVIII.13–15). This is reminiscent of the Egyptian myth where the lioness-headed goddess Sekhmet appears as "lady of the messenger of death"[49] and that Sekhmet is the goddess who could send epidemics upon man through her emissaries.[50] It may be an inference from Egyptian demonical aetiology. Throughout the medical papyri there is evidence for words which bear a determinative for "death" or "enemy" (Gardiner sign-list: A 14) or one of the determinatives for deities (e.g. Gardiner sign-list: G 7). Possibly these words refer to specific demons. Breasted (1930: 475) notices a general term for a disease-bearing demon, *ḫ3yty*, which is evidently derived from *ḫ3yt*, "disease," thus the "disease-demon."[51] Sometimes the name of a demon is specified, as in "son of the Disease-demon, *dnd*-demon" (Sm.verso.XVIII.1–8)[52]; the *srḫy*-demon is mentioned as "the leader of those who cause illness" (He.78). The *nsyt*-demon appears as an attacker of the belly (Eb.209) and the *ḥsk*-demon (lit. "the cutter") in the ear causes deafness (Eb.854e). These demons can be interpreted as the emissaries of Sekhmet, but it is not necessarily so. The causing of diseases by divine forces or by the deceased is directly indicated in the Egyptian medical texts that mention eye-diseases being caused "by a god, by dead man or by dead woman" (Eb.385), or a disease named *ʿ3ʿ* "by god and goddess" (Bln.58), "by god or a dead man" (Eb.225, 229) and "a dead man or woman" (Eb.99).

The *ʿ3ʿ* is a mysterious disease that appears several times in the medical papyri. It occurs 50 times in 4 papyri (28 in Ebers, 12 in Berlin, 9 in Hearst and once in London papyrus) (Ghalioungui 1973: 58). The description of its symptoms seems to relate it mainly to abdominal diseases, but it is quite difficult to identify the disease (see p. 33-4). Its curious relationships could relate not only to the god and the dead but also to the *ḥrrt*-worm (Eb.62) and an aetiological entity called *wḫdw* (Eb.138).

The *wḫdw* is very difficult word to understand. It is almost certainly related to the well-attested verb *wḫd* which means "to suffer" (Gardiner 1957: 562; Nunn 1996: 61), but it normally carries the determinative of pus (Gardiner sign-list: Aa 2). Ebbell (1937) translates it as "purulency," Grapow (1961: 207) and Westendorf (1999: 329) as "Schmerzstoffe" and Faulkner (1962: 68) as "pain." The textual studies of the *wḫdw* suggest that it is an aetiological agent related to faecal matter in the bowel that can cause various illnesses through its putrefaction power rather than being simply the name of a disease (see p. 32-3, 47). There are many terms that carry the pus determinative, and they appear to be aetiological agents or names of diseases such as *stt* (e.g. Eb.102), *w3šš* (Eb. 734), *3dt* (e.g. Eb.365) and *w3ḏ* (e.g. Eb.191). There are also other terms for symptoms or diseases that bear other kinds of determinatives such as the discharging phallus (Gardiner sign-list: D 53), and a sparrow (Gardiner sign-list: G 37). The examples of such disease terms are *fgn* (e.g. Eb.27), *ḥbdw* (Eb.265), *šmmt* (e.g. Eb.303), *gḥw* (Eb.326) and *ʿrwt* (e.g. Eb.857). Some of the disease terms are translatable as in the case of *ḥk3* ("magic"; e.g. Eb.165), *wnm* ("eater/ eating"; e.g. Eb.813), *wnm snf* ("blood eater/ blood eating"; e.g. Eb.722), *ʿ3t nt ḫnsw* ("Chons' swelling"; e.g. Eb.873) and *šʿt ḫnsw* ("Chons' cutting"; e.g. Eb.877).

[49] In "The destruction of mankind," the sun-god Ra set out to destroy the human race and the *sḫmt* ("Powerful One" i.e. Sekhmet) is sent out to slay mankind (Lichtheim 1976: 197–9).

[50] Pinch (1994: 37) notes that the Seven Arrows of Sekhmet always brought evil fortune, often in the form of infectious diseases. In "The tale of Sinuhe," Amunenshi, an Asiatic ruler, compared fear of the pharaoh Senusret I with that of "Sekhmet in a year of plague" (Lichtheim 1973: 225). At first Sekhmet was worshipped for fear of her wrath, but soon came to be considered as a benevolent healing deity, probably because it was argued that she who knew how to cause the disease also knew how to heal (Ghalioungui 1973: 14–5), and this could be the reason that the priests of Sekhmet were associated with medicine.

[51] Grapow (1962: 646) also translates as "Krankheitsdämon."

[52] Breasted (1930: 474) states that this term is the name of a demon doubtless derived from the old word *ḏnd* ("anger" or "wrath"), and he also notes that a disease term of similar phonetic value *ḏnḏ* in the Ebers papyrus (Eb.855v) is an ailment.

Egyptian pharmacopoeia

Around 500 words are employed for the medicinal materials in the Egyptian prescriptions, yet in most cases their identification remains uncertain or unclear.[53] Often the accompanying determinatives serve to indicate the nature of the materials such as plant or tree, animal (quadruped, bird, fish, snake), mineral or fruit and liquid substances, which can be helpful when considering at least the origins or nature of the materials (Westendorf 1999: 491). The Egyptian *materia medica* is commonly classified into categories of plant, animal and mineral origin.[54] The terms for materials also include the indications of parts or products obtained from their sources including seed, leaf, root and oil of a plant or meat, fat, blood and milk of an animal. Examples of processed products are beer, wine, honey and wax.[55] It appears that most of the materials employed throughout the Egyptian prescriptions are derived from the plant kingdom. But Germer (1993: 70) estimated that it was possible to identify only 20 per cent of some 160 plant products mentioned in the medical texts, and the diversity and disagreement in identifications among scholars has often led to further confusion of the situation.[56] In some cases, obscure expressions that do not disclose the composition of the material are used, such as *im twt* ("statue-clay"; Eb.511) and *ir-pt* ("heaven's eye" or "eye of the sky"; Eb.776) (see p. 40).

The Egyptian medical papyri do not provide us with explanatory statements concerning the pharmacological effect that Egyptians expected to obtain from the materials or the pharmacological principles by which they affirmed their efficacy. But there is one important exception, a text in the Ebers papyrus (Eb.251) that mentions the benefits of a plant called *dgm*:

> To know what is made with the *dgm*-plant as that which was found in old writings as something useful to men: Its roots are crushed in water and applied to a head which is ill, then he will get well immediately, like one who is not ill. But if a little of its seed is chewed with beer by a man with looseness in his excrements—it is an expulsion of the disease in the belly of a man. Further the hair of a woman is made to grow by means of its seed: it is ground, mixed together, and put into oil by the woman who shall rub her head herewith. Further oil of its seed is used to anoint one who (suffers) from *wḫ3w*, affected with *iṯṯt* and *ḥw3w*, which is painful. Then *rjwmw* come to a standstill like one to whom nothing has happened.[57] But he is treated by rubbing the aforesaid for 10 days, rubbing in very early in the morning, until it is expelled.

The identification of the *dgm*-plant is generally accepted as *Ricinus communis*. This plant is commonly known to us as the castor-oil plant. Grapow (1961: 203) takes *wḫ3w* to mean a skin disease ("Hautasschlag"; rash). Sigerist (1951: 340–1) points out that today castor-oil is a common ingredient in lotions for the scalp and ointments applied in the treatment of sores, and it is also used as a cathartic remedy.[58] This means we still use the plant for the same purposes as the Egyptians did, thus suggesting that the ancient Egyptians had proper knowledge of the pharmacological effects of this plant.[59]

Another genre of text that points to the pharmacological property that Egyptians assumed to be present in a material is the incantation which is to be recited with the administration of a remedy. For instance, the "milk of a woman who has born a male child" is strangely included as an ingredient in remedies for burns, but this substance is connected with the maternal goddess Isis who fed her son Horus. Since the goddess repeatedly helped her son in the Egyptian myth and healed Horus' burns, the incantations in the Ebers papyrus attached to remedies for burns is formulated "your son Horus is burnt in the desert. Is water there? There is no water there. There is water in my mouth and a Nile between (my) thighs. I came to extinguish the fire" (Eb.499) or in another place "my son Horus is burnt in the desert. There is no water there, I am not there. Bring you water from the shore and liquid to extinguish the fire" (Eb.500). Thus the mythical precedent for the healing property of milk established through association with the power of the goddess Isis.[60]

[53] Grapow and von Deines, *Wörterbuch der Drogennamen* list 500 remedies, and they give 358 translations as certain; 167 as doubtful or unidentified; and 19 illegible. Ebbell's translation of the Ebers papyrus includes 244 identifications, but it includes many tentative or questionable ones.

[54] For the materials that are commonly suggested as identifications, see the Appendix.

[55] Westendorf (1999: 514–5) provides the summary of the frequency distribution of terms referring to the different types of medicinal material and the condition in the medical papyri and notes "Bemerkenswert ist das Übergewicht der pflanzen, die mit über 40% den größten Anteil an den Drogen einnehmen."

[56] Nunn (1996: 152–4) provides lists showing the herbal substances with considerable agreement for the meaning of the Egyptian words and with less certain interpretation or alternative meanings attributed to the Egyptian word.

[57] Grapow (1961: 523) translates *rjwmw* as "krankhafte Erscheinung," and he notes that the text has been interpreted as *ʿḥʿ rwj mn.t* by Sander-Hansen, with *rjwm* being a misreading of *rwj mn.t*, i.e. "then the illness is removed."

[58] Jacob, I. (1993: 84) notes that eating as little as two seeds of this plant is fatal for children, as for adults 2–20 seeds cause coms and death in three days or less.

[59] Jacob, I. (1993) provides concise summary of medicinal use of the castor-oil plant in various places including ancient Egypt, Assyria, Greece, India and China as well as Europe in Middle Ages and modern societies. In it he notes, in modern chemotherapy, that castor oil is used as a cathartic, as a spermicide (vaginal jelly), against food poisoning, for clearing the bowels before X-ray examination, as a skin emollient, and as a solvent for removing irritating substances from the eye (Jacob, I. 1993: 86).

[60] This material is also used in the treatment for the *rš*-disease of the nose (Eb.763), and the accompanying incantation, which reads: "flow out, *rš* … I have brought you remedy against you … milk of a woman who has born a male child and fragrant gum; it expels you, it removes you," indicates its property of exorcism against the disease-entity.

3.3 Interpretation and comprehension of medical texts

The Egyptian medical texts can provide many important clues from which we can draw interpretations concerning the theoretical part of Egyptian medicine. On the one hand, an accurate reading of these texts requires a proper understanding of their lexicographical and philological basis and on the other, it is important to attempt to make proper interpretations in medical contexts, even though the texts of the Egyptian papyri, which include many difficult and uncertain terms, as well as the difficulties of medical anthropology, make it difficult to combine both approaches.

Egyptian pathology and aetiology

Diagnostic sign and disease-entity

There are many texts in the medical papyri describing symptomatic conditions and one also finds specific terms that may stand for a particular symptom, aetiological agent or disease. It is very important to understand that a significant difference exists between recognizing the meaning of a word and the symptom or disease itself. A symptom, in principle, is a mere phenomenon of abnormality, and it remains a symptom unless it is clinically interpreted. Then it becomes a diagnostic sign that conveys information indicative of a disease. This is indicative of the significant difference between a layman and physician. When a patient complains about the symptoms he is suffering from, it is the physician who is sufficiently proficient to recognize the diagnostic symptoms and reach a clinical conclusion identifying the pathological condition, pathogen or disease, while the layman cannot. A single symptom whose presence is directly connected to a particular pathogen or disease is called a pathognomonic symptom, but usually a single symptom alone such as a fever or a stomach-ache is inadequate to indicate a specific disease because these symptoms are indicative of many different ailments. But when symptoms occur in a cluster and form a coherent pattern, they can point toward a particular pathogen and disease (King 1982: 99). Thus, when we consider the disease terminology of the Egyptians to be the specific names of diseases rather than just the symptomatic expression, this means the Egyptian physicians actually succeeded in establishing a standardised nomenclature of disease by which a characteristic set of symptoms or a relevant pathogen was understood (Fig. 6).

Many scholars think the Egyptian "disease terms" are names of symptoms. Ebbell draws attention to the fact that in most cases, the Egyptians had names for simple symptoms only. If, therefore, the physicians referred to a more complicated disease not characterised by one single symptom, they had to give a description or write about "cases" as they are usually called (Temkin 1938: 126). But others assert the possibility of the Egyptians' having achieved a standardised nomenclature.[61] Ghalioungui (1966a: 127) writes:

> There is no concept more abstract or more elusive than that of disease. To primitive man, disease was a symptom. All archaic medical treatises are symptomatic pharmacopoeias. But as soon as the primitive mind started to work, it started to theorize, and nothing could then stop it in its accelerated course. The earliest grouping of symptoms to clearly defined syndromes, re-appearing with reasonable faithfulness to type, may have been a contribution of the Egyptian physicians who described, under the names of aaa, spn, skw.t, tmj.t. etc., certain symptom associations, although it is not clear from their writings whether these names defined the symptom-complex or the external agent to which disease was then attributed.

It is indeed difficult to say from the Egyptian writings whether the names represented symptoms or diseases. It is true that until relatively recently, confusion between the symptom and disease has been common among the medicines. King (1982: 161) notes that at one time, fever was regarded as a disease, and so also inflammation or

[61] Breasted (1930: 473) notes that there is no indication of the character of the disease "The pest of the year" found in the verso of the Edwin Smith papyrus, but it is characteristic of magical exorcism that there should be no proper examination, and no conclusions regarding the seat and the nature of the disease.

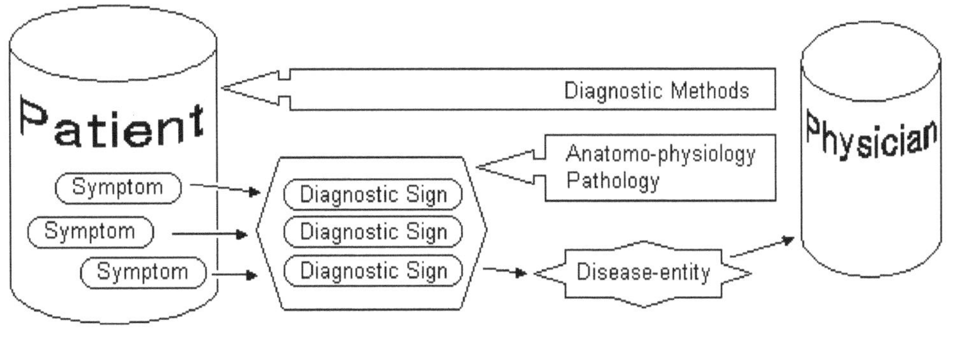

FIG. 6: DIAGNOSTIC PROCEDURE IN WHICH SYMPTOMS ARE REGARDED AS DIAGNOSTIC SIGNS POINTING TO A DISEASE-ENTITY.

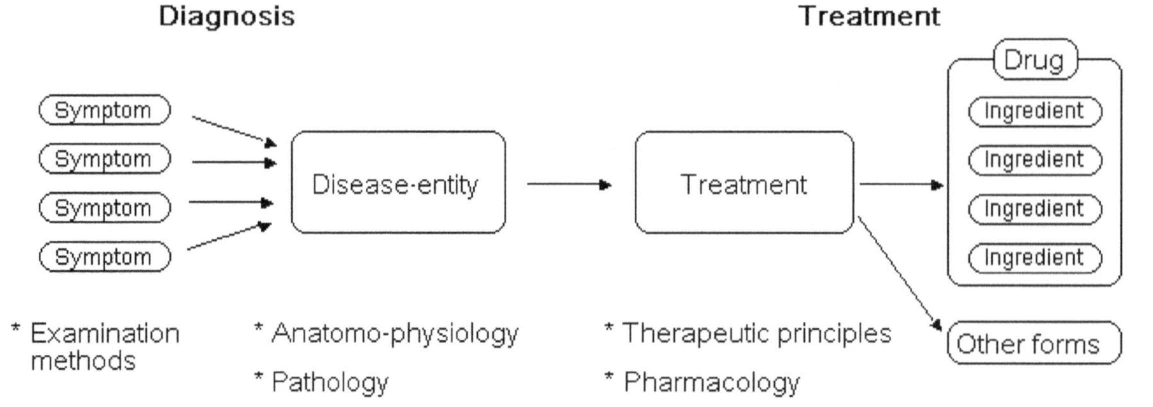

FIG. 7: THE APPLICATION OF EXPERT KNOWLEDGE IN THE PROCESS OF CLINICAL TREATMENTS.

jaundice, which are now purely regarded as symptoms. But it is necessary to emphasise that the study of Egyptian medical texts reveals the fact that the symptoms were regarded as important diagnostic criteria by the Egyptian, and they developed an understanding of disease based on the symptoms. As already mentioned, diagnosis is central to medical practice since it reveals the symptoms and leads to understanding of the disease.

A course of treatment is based on such an understanding (Fig. 7). Thus the essence of diagnosis is first to gather any diagnostic signs which require interpretation. Diagnostic signs would not be limited to apparent abnormalities and morbidities even those realized by the patient himself, but more often the physicians attentively use their expertise in diagnostic method to bring forth the diagnostic signs hidden in the inner parts of the body. An example of a diagnosis which can show the proficiency of the Egyptian physicians is the tactile observation of the pulse of a patient. An Egyptian text (Eb.854a; Bln.163; Sm.1) states that "any physician, any priest of Sekhmet or any magician applies his hands or his fingers to the (patient's) head, to the back of the head, to the hand, to the place of the heart (cardia), to the arms or to the feet, then he *ḫ3t* (examines) the heart because all his limbs possess its *mṯw*, that is: it (the heart) speaks out of *mṯw* of every limb." In the Egyptian anatomo-physiology, the heart is a central organ from which the *mṯw* are spread to the organs and body parts. The sentence "the heart speaks out of *mṯw* of every limb" is generally taken as the poetical expression for the pulse of blood-vessels that synchronises with the beat of the heart. Overall, this phrase would mean that the physicians were applying their fingers to the place of peripheral parts where the pulse can be felt. Regarding the manner of pulse examination by the ancient Egyptians, Breasted (1930: 105) considers that the physicians did count the pulse to observe the pulse rate. He explains that the word *ḫ3t* is used in the text to mean "examine," and the *ḫ3t* can be related to the well-known verb *ḫ3y* which means "to measure" used of grain, of area of land or of weighing, and this word in the medical texts could be conceived in the sense of counting. His opinion could be supported further by a gloss text attached to that paragraph which is only found in the Edwin Smith papyrus (Sm.1), which explains, "As for 'you *ḫ3t* (examine) a man' (it means) *ipt* (counting) any one … like counting things with a bushel. (For) examining is like one's counting a certain quantity with a bushel, (or) counting something with finger in order to (know) … one in whom an ailment is counted, like measuring the ailment of a man (and) of the heart." Breasted asserts the fact that the verb *ipt* which aptly means "to count" was employed to explain the word *ḫ3t* as if the text is emphasising measuring the pulse by counting.

However, to take pulse rate by counting the number of strokes requires an instrument which can measure very short periods of time accurately. The only such device in antiquity was the water-clock, and it was Herophilus of Alexandria of the Ptolemaic Period who appears to have been the first physician recorded in medical history to demonstrate the observation of the pulse rate by using a water-clock (*klepsydra*) (Nunn 1996: 207). Breasted (1930: 7–9) thinks that the pharaonic physicians might already have been practicing pulse examination in this same way. But some scholars are cautious of accepting his opinion. Ghalioungui (1973: 39) comments that it is not certain that water-clocks were in general use before the New Kingdom since only two water-clocks have so far been found which date back to the reigns of Thutmosis III and of Merneptah, and he states "if Breasted's supposition is confirmed, the author of the papyrus would have been far in advance of Hippocrates and Democritus who, 1000 years later, did not mention the rate of the pulse." Sigerist (1951: 330) notes that "even if the Egyptian had counted the pulse it could not have meant much to them since their knowledge of the cardio-vascular system was necessarily primitive."

This approach to understanding diagnostic examination by the pulse seems to be based on a modern medical understanding. Pulse examination is an important diagnostic method in Chinese and Āyurvedic medicine too, and these have attained extreme sophistication. The practitioners of Chinese medicine examine the rate of pulse beats with the time taken for them to complete an act of breathing, i.e. one inhalation and one exhalation (Ramachandra 1985: 50). The normal rate of pulse beat is considered to be four in one breathing. There are three kinds of pulse rate designated as "inch", "bar" and "cubit" (Wiseman 1995: 116). They are also skilled in feeling the pulse with a light touch or with some pressure, watching whether the pulse is superficial or deep, irregular, gentle or frisky, or even inner (*yin*) or outer (*yang*) pulse-let, and through the pulse examination they can detect disturbances and identify the related organs in which the disease originated (Ramachandra 1985: 50; Wiseman 1995: 116–21). Similarly, in Āyurvedic medicine, the form, mode, intensity and rhythmic frequency of the pulse are recognised by the physicians, and these can be understood with the association of their Three Humours Theory so that the pulse afflicted by *vata* takes an irregular or zigzag course, the pulse afflicted by *pitta* has a jumping motion like that of a frog, and the pulse afflicted by *kapha* is slow and moves like a swan (Warrier 1997: 128). A similar practice of pulse examination can be found in Galen who defines an abnormal pulse of excessive breath as "broad," of excessive length as "long" and of excessive depth as "deep," and in like manner the opposite of these as "narrow", "short" and "shallow" (Clendening 1960: 42–3).[62] Thus, it is not farfetched to assume that the ancient Egyptian physicians could recognise features of the pulse and regarded them as clues to understanding disease just as Galen did and the Chinese and Indian physicians do through the application of their own medical theories.[63]

Also noteworthy is the common trend to associate blood vessels with breath or air found in the different medicines. In a text of the Ebers papyrus (Eb.855a) the cardiological function of the heart, lung and *mṯw* is mentioned: "as to the breath/air which enters into the nose. It enters into the heart and lung. It is they (*mṯw*) which give (breath/air) to the entire body." This may surprise us because the substitution of the word "air" with "oxygen" makes the whole concept close to the truth (Nunn 1996: 55). Breasted (1930: xvi) considers that the Egyptian "was surprisingly near recognition of the circulation of the blood, for he was already aware that the heart was the center and the pumping force of a system of distributing vessels." This opinion is often taken as over-enthusiastic, for the actual discovery of blood circulation requires detailed observation methods and profound biological knowledge. Nonetheless, it is interesting that the Egyptian text (Eb.855e) mentions "As to 'faintness' it is that the heart does not speak or the *mṯw* of the heart are dumb, there being no perception of them under your fingers."

Chinese anatomo-physiology describes the distribution of blood and breath through 12 channels of the body (or 14 according to some) (Ramachandra 1985: 51). In a curious coincidence we find the Ebers papyrus (Eb.856b) has a passage that mentions "As to man, there are 12 *mṯw* to his heart. It is they which give to all his limbs." The parallel passage in the Berlin papyrus (Bln.163b), however, contains a different figure "... 22 *mṯw* in him. They draw off air to his heart. It is they which give breath/air to each of his two arms." It is considered that the number twelve in the Ebers papyrus is a scribal error since the figure of twenty-two in the Berlin papyrus is the exact total for *mṯw* in the Ebers (Eb.856) and Berlin (Bln.163) papyrus combined (Nunn 1996: 48).

Faecal pathology

Kutumbiah (1957: 17) points to a particular similarity in the concept of vessels between the ancient Egyptian and Āyurvedic medicine through the comparative study of the notion of *mṯw* in the Egyptian texts and that of vessels held in *Samhitās* of *Charaka* and *Suśruta* (6th century BC). According to him, the Charaka (C.S.III 5. 2–16) describes the vessels that carry the force of life-breath to the heart, and they also serve as passages carrying water and food, chyle and blood, and transformations of the latter, namely, fat, bone, marrow and semen as well as urine, excrements and sweat (17). But the vessels relate to the humours of *vata*, *pitta* and *kapha* that are unique to India. The description of specific functions of vessels shows that some are connected with the place of *pitta* and they draw downwards the material not fit to be absorbed, and they nourish the body as soon as it is digested by the action of heat, by supplying it to the upper circulatory vessels and through them to the heart, which is designated as the seat of *rasa-sthana* (17).

Kutumbiah (1957: 13) emphasises that "the resemblance is very striking when we consider the role of the vessels in the production of disease ... when these vessels grow irritated, the constituents of the body grow irritated. The irritation spreads from one kind of vessel to the others. Vessels harm vessels, so constituents harm constituents, when irritated." Actually some inferences about the relationship between the *mṯw* and disease can be found in the Egyptian medical texts. Eb.854l states "There are 4 *mṯw* to the liver. It is they which gives to it water and breath/air, which afterward cause all diseases to appear in it through overfilling with blood." Another text (Eb.855v) states "As to 'A whirl has fallen on his heart.' This means that a whirl of *t3w*-heat has fallen on his heart. This is frequent weakness. This means that he becomes powerless as a result of *ḏnḏ*. It is the

[62] Galen wrote in several treatises on the pulse including *Libellus de Pulsibus ad Tirone, Libri Quatuor de Pulsum Differentiis, Libri Quatuor de Pulsibus Dignoscendis, Libri Quatuor de Causis Pulsuum, Libri Quatuor de Praesagitione ex Pulsibus, Synopsis Sexdecim Librorum de Pulsibus* and *Pulsuum Compendium* (Clendening 1960: 42).

[63] Dominique Spaeth, in his doctoral thesis, argues that the Egyptian physicians examined the pulse "qualitatively (in terms of strength and rhythm) and semi-quantitatively (slow or accelerated), though the writings so far discovered do not mention this" (quoted in Halioua 2005: 25). Also Stephan (2005: 89) states "Über 1000 jahre bevor etwas Ähnliches in der griechischen Medizin nachweisbar ist, haben wir es hier zu tun mit einer Pulslehre, und zwar einer Pulslehre, die den Schlag des Herzen nicht nur qualitative in Beziehung setzt zur Krankheit des Patienten, sondern die diese Krankheit quantitative nach Zahl und Maß zu erfassen versucht, wie die naturwissenschaftliche Medizin unserer Tage."

fullness of his heart with blood that does it. It arises through drinking water, (and) eating hot *sbj*-fish is what causes it to arise." Also Eb.855f reads "As to 'his heart is bored.' It is (due to) his heart is weak because of heat of the anus. You find it large, things rolling in his stomach like *s(j) m ir.t* (lit. "she in the eye": i.e. iris?)." In the Egyptian medical texts, it is very difficult to make precise interpretations of the pathological concepts expressed, but it is evident in the Egyptian theory of anatomo-physiological pathology where the diseases emerge due to abnormal conditions of organs or malfunction of the *mṯw*. It is also noticeable that the Egyptian pathology also takes the dietetic causes into account, as we find in the case of eating hot *sbj*-fish that leads to disease.

The Egyptian medical texts occasionally refer to faecal matter in the bowel as an aetiological agent. Eb.856h says that "all together (*mṯw*) go to his heart, divide to his nose, all together (*mṯw*) unite to his hinder part, and illness of the hinder part arises through them (*mṯw*), and it is faeces that are carried, it is (*mṯw*) of the feet that begin to die." We can also find a text (Eb.855g) which mentions "As to 'His heart spread itself out.' It is that the *mṯw* of the heart are carrying faeces." This indication of the concept of faecal pathology is reminiscent of the records of Herodotus and Diodorus. Herodotus (II, 77) reports on the practice of medicine that he observed during this travel to Egypt that "for three successive days in each month they purge, hunting after health with emetics and clysters, and they think that all the disease which exist are produced in men by the food on which they live" (trans. Macaulay 1904: 150). A similar report is provided by Diodorus (I, 82), who writes "in order to prevent sickness they look after the health of their bodies by means of drenches, fasting, and emetics, sometimes every day and sometimes at intervals of three or four days. For they say that the larger part of the food taken into the body in superfluous and that it is from this superfluous part that diseases are engendered; consequently the treatment just mentioned, by removing the beginnings of disease, would be most likely to produce health" (trans. Oldfather 1933: 281). These records both make mention of the fact that the Egyptians considered that the residue from food in the bowel was a cause of disease, and to prevent disease and maintain health they regularly practiced evacuations to remove morbid faecal matter from the body. These statements actually accord well with the fact that there are many evacuation treatments contained in the Egyptian medical papyri. We can also find direct indications of the Egyptian notion of faecal pathology in the titles of prescriptions such as, "to expel noxious excrements in the belly of a man" (Eb.30) and "to empty the belly and make all evil that is in the body of a man come out" (Eb.22). Thus we may speculate that the Egyptian evacuation practices that Herodotus and Diodorus witnessed were practices based on a faecal pathological theory that had already existed in Egypt for at least 1000 years before their visit.

With regard to the origin of faecal pathology in Egypt, it is generally considered as being related to the observation of decomposition in corpses. Putrefaction after death is characterized by heat and odour initially from the bowels which then spreads to all organs, and eventually corruption of the entire body occurs. From observation of this fact, together with the characteristic heat and disagreeable smell after evacuation, ancient people may have assumed putrefaction of faecal residue in the bowel possessed a destructive power. An Egyptological interpretation has been made through associations with the mummification tradition of Egypt. The essence of mummification practice is the removal of the bowels to prevent putrefaction and destruction of the corpse, and it is, in a sense, a therapeutic procedure for the corpse. This view is supported by the fact that the Egyptian word *sdwḫ* has the meaning "to embalm" in the Book of the Dead and "to treat" in the medical texts (Steuer *et al.* 1959: 2; Saunders 1963: 23).[64] There may be some connection between the Egyptian practices of diagnostic observation of the patient's stool with the notion of faecal pathology. We can find medical texts which give instructions, following the application of the first treatments, to examine the course of the treatment by observing if the substances "that have gone out of his anus like broken particles (?) of beans, and dew runs out like a flow of *tp3w.t*" (Eb.207), or "that comes in this case from his mouth or his anus like swine's blood after it is fried" (Eb.198) and also the observation of "what is lifted by cough (i.e. phlegm)" (Eb.190).

Nevertheless, faecal pathology is a very common pathological theory seen in many different medicines including Greek, Chinese and Indian medicine.[65] It is also evident in the medicine of a culture that does not have a mummification tradition. Sometimes considerable similarity is evident in the theories of faecal pathology. But here as well, it is difficult to tell if this pathology has a single origin, which spread through cultural associations, or whether it consists of endogenous occurrences of similar concepts in different places. But it is also true that there are significant differences among the medicines, and thus we can not make simple comparisons. For instance, the Āyurvedic diagnosis of excreta where the stool is hard, dry, rough and of a garish colour is considered being aggravation by *vata*; a greenish and liquid stool being by *pitta*, and whitish stool mixed with mucus being by *kapha* (Warrier 1997: 129).

Disease terminology

A concept of faecal pathology peculiar to the ancient Egyptians seems to be represented by the disease term *wḫdw*. This term appears in the medical papyri relatively frequently compared to other disease terms. The study of the contexts suggests that the *wḫdw* is associated with faecal matter as we can compare the titles of the prescriptions

[64] Erman (1953: 368) states that *sdwḫ* in the sense of "treat" is identical with *srwḫ*, and Grapow (1962: 775) lists *sdwḫ* with *srwḫ*. The confusion is probably due to the similarity of *r* and *d* in hieratic.

[65] See p. 47 for a discussion of the Greek faecal pathology.

with sections referring to evacuation treatment that mention "Another to empty the belly and make all evil that is in the body of a man come out" (Eb.22), "Another to expel noxious excrement in the belly of a man" (Eb.30) and "Another to empty the belly and expel *wḫdw* in the belly of a man" (Eb.32). Also, in another section "Another to expel *wḫdw* in the belly" or to "clear out *wḫdw*" (e.g. Eb.86, 87, 97, 98). One may interpret the *wḫdw* as a specific aetiological agent that emerges from the faecal residue. It is quite difficult, however, to understand the precise nature of the *wḫdw* from the study of the texts. It can occur not only in abdominal parts and the anus (Eb.141) but also in the heart (Eb.855m), eye (Eb.341), mouth (Eb.122), gum (Eb.741) and jugular region (Eb.187). The symptoms caused by *wḫdw* vary so that the presence of the *wḫdw* "on his heart" causes "senile decay (*wj3wj.t*)" (Eb.855m) and "the heart kneels down because of the *wḫdw*" (Eb.855l). Sometimes the *wḫdw* appears in wounds as in a remedy "to heal wound when *wḫdw* arise" (Eb.130) and in "*ḥnḥn.t*-ulcer that has appeared through an attack of *wḫdw*" (Eb.858). The putrefaction power of the *wḫdw* is evident when we see the *wḫdw* apparently being used in the sense of "pus," as we can compare the texts "swelling of pus" (Eb.869) and "swelling of *wḫdw*" (Eb.871). We may notice the analogy between the heat involved in the putrefaction of the bowel and the inflammation of swelling.[66]

In four places (Eb.131, 242, 246, 385), the word *wḫdw* appears with the feminine termination as *wḫdwt*, alongside the *wḫdw* as if it has a separate identify from *wḫdw*, but the difference between them remains unclear. There are several more terms that can be understood in a similar way to the *wḫdw*, but due to their lower frequency of occurrence in the medical papyri and an insufficient number of texts to consult, their interpretation also remains uncertain.[67] One such term is the *stt* which also carries the pus determinative, but in two cases it also carries the water determinative 𓈗 (Gardiner sign-list: N 35), which may imply its liquid nature.[68] The putrefaction nature related to the faecal residue of the *stt* is indicated in a text which reads "If you examine one who suffers from *stt* from *nkʿw.t* (cutting?) and whose belly is stiff through it, and he suffers in his stomach. When his *stt* is in his belly, and it does not find a way to come out, nor is there (any) way by which it can come out, then it shall rot in his belly, and being able to come out, it grows into a *ḥsb.t*" (Eb.102 = 296). Another diagnostic text (Eb.192) mentions "If you examine one who suffers in his stomach and vomits (*ḳ3s*) frequently. If you find it being in front of him, both his eyes are inflamed (*šsm*) and his nose runs (*tḫb*). Then you should say, 'These are putrefactive (*sḫw3w*) products of his *stt*, they could not go down' " (Eb.192 = 195). In most cases the treatment of the *stt* is evacuation (e.g. Eb.102, 192). Also, the *ʿrwt* which appears in four cases in the Ebers papyrus can be understood as an etiological entity of this kind (Eb.207, 857, 859, 862).

Another disease term frequently discussed is the *wnm snf* (e.g. Eb.749). This is also a very difficult term to interpret as it can yield different understandings. Grapow (1958: 243) translates it as "Blutfressen" (blood eating) and Westendorf (1999: 356) translates it as "Blut-fraß," taking it as a verbal sentence as if the *snf* itself is the pathogenic agency.[69] Contrary to Grapow, Lefebvre (1956) conceives it syntactically as an infinitive and translates it as "mangeur de sang" (blood eater) suggesting a pathogenic agency which eats up the blood.[70] Some scholars attempt to provide identifications of this disease from contextual interpretation and suggestions include "pyorrhea" by Lefebvre (1956) and "scurvy" by Ebbell (1937) and Leake (1952). Nonetheless the pathological concept of the *wnm snf* remains obscure.

The *ꜥ3ʿ* is a curious disease term that has received considerable documentation. The identification of this term is suggested by Ebbell (1937: 35) as the haematuria resulting from schistosomiasis, the infection of the parasitic worm Bilharzia. The three main points that lead to this identification are (1) throughout the papyri the *ꜥ3ʿ* is almost invariably qualified by the adjective "deadly," (2) the *ꜥ3ʿ* is related to the *ḥrrw*-worm (Eb.62), and (3) the term carries the discharging phallus as determinative which could be seen as representing bloody urine (Hussein 1998: 61). The text (Eb.62) which plays a significant role in the identification is:

> Another excellent remedy amongst those prepared for the belly: *isw*-plant 1, *šʿms*-plant 1, are ground fine, boiled with honey and eaten by a man in whose belly there are *ḥrrw*-worms. It is the *ꜥ3ʿ* that produced them. Not killed by any (other) remedy.

Ebbell (1937: 35) provides a footnote concerning the *ḥrrw*-worms linking "By this Bilharzia haematobia must no doubt be meant, a trematode worm, which is found in the veins of the abdominal organs in the haematuria which is endemic in Egypt." Jonchkeere (1944) supports this identification. According to him, the *ꜥ3ʿ* can be clinically

[66] For Egyptian disease description of *wḫdw* and its related diseases and body parts, see Grapow (1961: 207–17) and Westendorf (1999: 341–3); Westendorf (1999: 330–41) presents the prescriptions against *wḫdw* in the medical papyri.

[67] Through a reconsideration of the difficult term *wḫdw*, Kolta *et al.* (2000: 52) conclude "Accordingly, we propose the following hypotheses: *wḫdw* designates causes of illness or pathogenic agents in a rather unspecific way. It may refer to all kinds of disease agents which will spread all over the human body through the vascular system. An adequate German rendering of the term could be 'Leidensmacher'."

[68] Westendorf (1999: 343) translates *stt* as "Schleimstoffe," noting that it is based on the "Verbum *stj* 'strömen, gießen' " and also the water determinative (Eb 102 und 206a). The circulation of the *stt* in the body is observed: "Es sind also Stoffe, die im Körper umherziehen (*ḥtḥt* Bln 138) oder sich in bestimmte Körperteile 'ergießen' (*stj* Sm 43 [15,5]) Können, und zwar an allen beliebigen Stellen (Bln 136, 139, 140) oder 'im Fleisch des Mannes' (Bln 138). Sie ähneln in dieser Hinsicht den Schmerzstoffen, als deren Weg durch den Körper eindeutig das Gefäßsystem genannt ist (Eb 856a = Bln 163a)" (Westendorf 1999: 343); Bardinet (1995: 125) notes the *stt* as "êtres pathogens circulants."

[69] Westendorf (1999: 356) notes that "Anders als im koptischen ⲟⲩⲁⲙ-ⲥⲛⲟϥ 'Blut-Fresser' ist hier also das Blut der aktive Teil der Verbindung, d.h.es liegt ein Genitivus subiectivus vor."

[70] For detailed discussion on the *wnm snf*, see Steuer (1961).

characterized by abdominal distension, abdominal pain, palpitations, stitches, "escape" of the heart and blood-stained evacuation (Ghalioungui 1973: 58). Lefebvre (1956) and some other scholars follow this identification. But this identification has also been questioned. Ghalioungui (1973: 58–9) points out that it rests on an extremely bold hypothesis. Among fifty prescriptions and magical formula mentioning the *ꜥꜣꜥ*, there is only one that includes a worm, and the association with a blood-stained evacuation is deduced from the presence, in the middle of a few prescriptions against bleeding in the London papyrus, of a formula meant to treat *ꜥꜣꜥ* (Lo.13, 3–7). Ghalioungui comments that "If we accept these two flimsy arguments, we have, moreover, to believe that the Ancient Egyptians discovered the bilharzia worm that is only 1cm long, and 1 or 2 mm thick, that lives hidden in the deep veins in the abdomen, and that undergoes autolysis 24 hours after death," and in support of his criticism he quotes Grapow (1956: 65): "How could the Egyptians have discovered this very small worm, and what would have suggested to them the idea of a connection between it and haematuria?"[71] Indeed, it would be unfounded to identify the *ꜥꜣꜥ* as the haematuria.[72] As a further argument, we can also note that there are several prescription texts that mention blood-stained evacuation (e.g. Eb.49; Bln.165), and while these might be a result of the haematuria, none of these mention the *ꜥꜣꜥ*. Also from modern medicine we know that a bloody evacuation is not a pathognomonic symptom that is immediately connected to bilharziasis.

In some passages we find a curious aspect of *ꜥꜣꜥ*-disease, where the Egyptian texts indicate its association with supernatural entities such as "to expel *ḥkꜣ* (magic?) and *ꜥꜣꜥ* of a god or dead man" (Eb.168). With this feature in mind Grapow (1961: 129–31) proposed a different, Egyptological interpretation of this disease, which is concisely summarized by Nunn (1996: 63):

> Their concept was essentially that of an evil spirit in the form of an incubus who impregnated its victims with its poisonous semen while they were asleep ... This is supported by the fact that there is a rare verb, *aaa* with the same determinative, which means 'to discharge semen.' Furthermore, many of the remedies against *aaa* are to be taken at night when an incubus would be most active. Therefore, *aaa* appears to be a poisonous and toxic substance introduced into the body by magical means, and was considered to be the cause of a variety of disease to be treated with remedies as well as incantation.

Grapow (1961: 132) mentions "daß es sich weniger um eine Krankheit, als um einen Krankheitsstoff handelt, der von Dämonen (Gespenstern oder bösen Göttern) in den Bauch des Patienten gebracht ist ..." Also Westendorf (1999: 361) notes that "Der Befall des Patienten erfolgte in der Nacht, der Dämon wird als ein Incubus angesehen, der die Menschen mit seinem Giftsamen schwängert." Therefore, it may be justifiable to attribute to it the meaning of "poisonous semen" of a demonical entity.[73] This would enable us to make sense of Bardinet's translation (1995: 416) of an Egyptian "Remède pour chasser le âaâ provenant d'un dieu, d'une déesse, la semence provenant d'un mort ou d'une morte" (Bln.58). Nevertheless, further confusions emerge when we read the Egyptian texts " to clear out *wḫdw* and expel *ꜥꜣꜥ* of a dead man or dead woman" (Eb.99) or "to expel *ꜥꜣꜥ* in a man, clear out *wḫdw*, (and) expel evil that appears in a man" (Eb.138), a curious combination of the *ꜥꜣꜥ* and the *wḫdw* (Westendorf 1999: 329).

Cultural aspects of the concept of disease

The interpretations of Egyptian medical terms are necessarily fragmentary and uncertain, and the Egyptian diagnostic text always disconnectedly reaches the diagnosis without a clear explanation for it.[74] And this has resulted in diverse interpretations which hardly allow us to comprehend the whole idea of the text. We do not know what is happening in the nose injury where "the clotting of blood inside of his two nostrils, likened to the *ꜥnꜥrt*-worm which lives in the water" (Sm.12), or what the incantation for "a man who has swallowed a fly" (Sm.verso.XIX. 14–8) can mean. Breasted (1930: 470, 482) gives a comment that the fly could have been a carrier of disease for the Egyptians as it can actually transmit diseases like dysentery. In the case of another incantation to prevent asses and a kind of goose from entering (Sm.verso.XIX. 12), however, it will be difficult to take such an animal as a carrier of disease. Ghalioungui (1973: 55) considers the fly, ass, goose and the like may all have been metaphorical expressions for demonical entities. There is a curious injury mentioned in the Edwin Smith papyrus namely "a smash in his skull under the skin of his head, there being no wound at all upon it" (Sm.8). This injury is diagnosed for "one whom something entering from outside has smitten," and the gloss attached to this paragraph explains "As for 'something entering from outside,' it means the wind/air of an outside god or dead; not the intrusion of something which his flesh engenders."

[71] Westendorf (1992: 253) notes "Hier an die winzigen Schistosoma zu denken, hieße den Ägyptern wahrhaft mikroskopische Fähigkeiten zuzutrauen."

[72] Westendorf (1999: 471), nevertheless, keeps this identification as a possible case that: "Bei den mehrschichtigen Krankheitsbildern der Bilharzia und *ꜥꜣꜥ*-Krankheit ist es jedoch durchaus möglich, daß einzelne Symptome der Bilharzia sich mit denen der *ꜥꜣꜥ*-Krankheit überschneiden, die Identifizierung also partiell denkbar ist."

[73] Concerning the discharging phallus determinative of *ꜥꜣꜥ*, Westendorf (1992: 252–3) states "Tatsächlich handelt es sich aber um das Wort für Samen bzw. Gift, das ein Incubus-Dämon nachts in den Menschen senkt. Also genau umgekehrt ist die Zielrichtung des Phallus: er führt Gift in den Leib des Menschen, nicht aber Harn und Blut als Ausscheidung aus ihm heraus!"

[74] The diagnostic text of Eb.192, for example, states "If you examine someone who suffers in his stomach and *kꜣs* (vomits) frequently; if you find it (disease) being in front of him, both his eyes are *šsm* (inflamed) and his nose *tḫb* (runs). Then you should say: These are *sḫwꜣ* of his *stt*: (they) could not go down to his *npḥw* as his *stt*."

We can assume the existence of a faecal pathological theory in ancient Egypt and can roughly understand the concept of specific putrefaction agencies such as *wḫdw* or *stt* that emerge from the faecal residue and spread into different parts of the body through the network of the *mṯw* in which various symptoms or even the transformation of pus occurs. But we do not understand properly the text "if you examine someone with an obstruction of his stomach, (and) he vomit very painfully, (and) he suffers from it as (from) *sḫ.t*, you shall say, this is a *ṯ3w* of faeces that has not yet attached itself" (Eb.202). Similarly we do not understand the pathological condition of the liver which is overfilled with blood (Eb.854l) or the heart suffering from heat from the anus (Eb.855f).

These Egyptian descriptions of diseases are very difficult to interpret and can hardly make sense to us. It is, however, very important to be aware that these descriptions were totally rational and understandable to the ancient Egyptians. An article by Lesile (1976: 225) discusses the particular communication problem that occurs between a local patient and a practitioner of modern medicine in Sri Lanka today, and may be helpful in understanding the situation:

> The language by which the patient describes symptoms is perfectly comprehensible to the Āyurvedic doctor, since it is derived from Āyurveda. Thus, patients establish communication and rapport with Āyurvedic physicians that are sadly lacking in interactions with Western doctors ... consider the following typical statements by patients suffering from dhātu loss: "Blood is heated and passes out," "the dhātu set heated and passed out" similarly, a patient may say that a serious headache is because "wind has struck the top"—i.e., an excess of wind produced in the region of the stomach has moved toward the reign of the head.

This means the patient uses the disease terms particular to Āyurvedic medicine and also describes his disease in ordinary words, but based on specific Āyurvedic medical concepts. It seems we are confronting a similar situation when we read the Egyptian medical text. Our insufficient lexicographical knowledge of the Egyptian disease terms and the totally different outlook on diseases lead us into confusion much like the problem encountered by practitioners of modern medicine in Sri Lanka. But just as the Āyurvedic doctors can perfectly comprehend the ailment described by a patient, the Egyptian medical texts must have been totally comprehensible to the ancient Egyptian physicians. We may even assume that the descriptions of the diseases in the medical papyri might have been expressions that could be understood by ordinary people in ancient Egypt as is suggested by a statement in a non-medical text, e.g. Ramesside text Papyrus Anastasi IV which reads "... A *mns*-scribe is here with me, every muscle of whose face twitches, the *wštt*-disease had developed in his eye and the *fnṯ*-worm[75] into his tooth. I cannot leave him to his fate ..." (Weeks 1980: 110; Westendorf 1999: 103).

Medicine, therefore, is an integrated component of cultural beliefs, and in order to understand the medicine of a particular culture we have to place it within the medical context of that culture. Is it then possible to ascertain how effective the interpretations of Egyptian medical texts are according to modern medical conceptions? Some scholars make enthusiastic attempts to identify the Egyptian diseases described in the medical papyri according to modern medical conceptions and try to apply our equivalent disease terms or the corresponding recognition of pathology. Ebbell's (1937) translation has often been criticised because he includes identifications and interpretations of the Egyptian diseases that are heavily reliant on modern concepts of disease, often with scant evidence. There are many identifications of Egyptian diseases established through interpretation based on a modern medical sense, but they are mostly questionable. Sometimes we find interpretations that go beyond what appears to be acceptable. It has, for example, been suggested that the Egyptian *wnmt m ḥmt* ("eater/eating in the womb") is a cancer (Ebbell 1928: 73) or the *ꜥ3ꜥ*-disease associated with Ebora-virus or HIV (Richard 1996: 242). We can consider such interpretations as highly speculative and improbable because they may not be applicable to the medical concepts of antiquity.

Difficulties in the interpretation of disease due to differences of culture can also appear even in the approach towards similar or identical terms. For instance, the term "wind" or "air" is commonly found associated with an evil epidemic disease among different cultures. In Japanese, the word for a cold (風邪) has the same phonetic value as wind "kaze" and consists of two characters representing wind (風) and evil (邪). Ghalioungui (1973: 53) mentions that today we use expressions such as "the flu is in the air," or "a sick person has caught wind or a cold." These are comparable to the Egyptian statement of "his flesh caught wind" (Sm.31),[76] but there can be significant differences in their pathological theories.

A significant difference in the concept of demonical-disease which exists between the Egyptian and the Semitic and Indo-European civilizations is the theological connotation in medicine whereby the concept of disease is regarded as a punishment for sin. Apparently the Sumerians frequently regarded illness as a punishment for sins. Hindu culture

[75] Westendorf (1999: 400) notes that this worm is probably "kein Eingeweide-Wurm" but rather "eine Erscheinung, die bei Nagel-Erkrankungen auftritt, wie durch H 196 erweisbar ist (Herausholen des fnt-Wurmes aus dem Finger {oder} der Zehe)."

[76] Ghalioungui (1967a: 40) also notes that this is "une expression qui rappelle, modestement il est vrai, les traités grecs sur les vents" and also "ceci correspond à la croyance populaire égyptienne que l'on est malade parce qu'on a «pris de l'air» اخد هوا ou un coup d'air لفمة هوا ou qu'un melon laissé toute une nuit coupe est malsain parce qu'il a «pris de l'air»."

possesses the notion of *Karma* which is the effect of good and evil deeds done in former lives or in this life that would bring one happiness or suffering including diseases during a later existence.[77] There are many Egyptian words denoting evil acts, but it appears more likely they should be taken to mean misdeed or aberrations, rather than sins (Frankfort 1961: 73).[78]

We cannot, therefore, expect to find medical terms of precise equivalence and translate one medical system into another language or culture completely. I would also point out that the meaning of medical terms is always subjected to change through time because physicians who developed or borrowed new medical ideas could devise a new term, but more often they applied old terms in a new sense. For example, the term "influenza" is originally related to "influence (of environment)," especially of the stars (Skeat 1901: 261; King 2001: 22), but now we use the term to refer to the concept of viral infection.

On the whole, the study of Egyptian medical texts reveals a richness of medical terminology that indicates the Egyptians' detailed understanding of the human body and its diseases. The diagnostic texts clearly reflect the depth of thought taken by physicians during clinical examination as well as the existence of pathological concepts shared by physicians, although the precise theory may not be comprehensible to us. A further significant fact that reveals the depth of practice and knowledge of Egyptian medicine is the inclusion of prognosis in the medical writings. The Edwin Smith papyrus regularly presents three cases of prognosis expressed by stock phrases that "an ailment which I will treat" (i.e. certainly treatable) (e.g. Sm.1), "an ailment with which I will contend" (i.e. possibly curable) (e.g. Sm.4) and "an ailment not to be treated" (i.e. hopeless and untreatable) (e.g. Sm.5). We can find the former two cases in the Ebers papyrus in the section on the treatment of trauma (Eb.857–62), and the prognosis for the *w3ḏ*-disease of the stomach states "it is death that threatens him" (Eb.191). These prognoses are an indication of the Egyptian physician's ability to foretell the possibility of recovery and convalescence. King (1982: 165) comments on the prognoses in antiquity that until relatively recently, since physicians could not do much to affect disease directly, when the laity tried to evaluate the merits of a physician, an important criterion was his ability to foretell what would happen, and hence if he could predict accurately, his reputation would rise. The most impressive prognosis shown in the medical papyri is the text, "moor (him) at his mooring stakes until the period of his injury passes by," and, in the gloss, the meaning of this metaphoric expression is explained "it means putting him on his customary diet without administering to him a prescription" (e.g. Sm.3), and the entire concept is clarified by a text "until you know that he has reached a decisive point" (e.g. Sm.4). This concept is comparable to the Hippocratic notion of the critical days. The gloss text that refers to the "decisive point" explains that "it means (until) you know whether he will die or he will live" (Sm.4).

Egyptian pharmacology

The empirico-rational element

The only material, in the medical papyri, whose medicinal efficacy is clearly stated, is the castor-oil plant (*dgm*) (Eb.251) (see p. 28), and Egyptian knowledge about the remaining hundreds of medicinal substances that were involved in prescriptions remains quite unclear. In principle, the pharmacological treatment is based on the knowledge and theory of disease. We may roughly posit three possibilities for Egyptian disease terms that are unclear to us—(1) the symptom which was primarily regarded as the disease, (2) the aetiological entity that causes disease and (3) the symptom and cause are conclusively understood and recognised by name. It follows that differences will appear in the assumptions underlying the intended treatment. If the symptom was being treated, the remedy might be designed for relief. If the aetiological agency is targeted in order to be eliminated, the remedy needs an ability to combat and expel the agency. So, employing a magical substance against demonical disease may be logical. If the disease was identified based on a particular pathological theory, a particular pharmacological theory applied may be in the treatment.

It is tempting to assume that the Egyptian physicians used their knowledge of the castor-oil plant in a purgative remedy "to empty the belly and expel *wḫdw*" (Eb.25) and in an ointment for a skin disease of the scalp (Eb.437). But the Egyptian pharmacological principle remains poorly understood, and our present understanding is generally based on the notion of primitive empirico-rational and magico-religious medicine. This may not be appropriate because when we consider the indications and features in the established conceptualisation of anatomo-physiology and pathology revealed by the medical texts and the Egyptian diagnoses in which the physicians follow a logical thought-process to identify a disease through diagnostic observational methods, then it appears probable there may also have existed well conceptualised pharmacological principles that were developed and shared by the Egyptian physicians and which extended beyond primitive empiricism and simple recognitions of magical property.

It is true, the application of an empirico-rational and magico-religious perspective can help us to formulate some hypothetical understandings of the principles of Egyptian pharmacology. The empirico-rational aspect of Egyptian pharmacology, it is suggested, is based on

[77] *Caraka* (iii.3.29–30) strongly emphasizes this concept (Basham 1976: 22).

[78] Ockinga (2001: 485) states that the term *isft*, which is usually translated "sin" or "wrong," designates a concept diametrically opposed to *m3ʿt*, as is seen as early as the Pyramid Texts (section 265), and an expression of *isft* as antonym of *m3ʿt* is also found in the Book of Going Forth by Day (ch.126). He notes that although *isft* is used in that text as an all-embracing term for "wrong," in ancient Egypt there was no concept of "general sin," a barrier between humankind and the gods which is the result of the general human condition.

the modern chemotherapeutic principle. One can point, for example, to the use of the strong laxative effect of colocynth or senna in the evacuation remedies (e.g. Eb.11), of the liver of ox, which is rich in vitamin A, for night blindness (Eb.351), of the strong antiseptic effect of salicin obtained from a decoction of willow leaves for wounds (e.g. Sm.41), of tannic acid, which is contained in the gallnuts of acacia and tamarisk, for burns (e.g. Eb.482), of the diuretic, stimulant and carminative effect of juniper berry for urinary disorders (e.g. Eb.263) and for evacuation (e.g. Eb.85; He.59), and of alkaloids (mainly of pelletierine) in the root of pomegranate as a vermifuge (Eb.50, 63).[79]

There has been much discussion among scholars about the Egyptian use of opium.[80] There is a disagreement among the scholars as to whether the Egyptians had access to opium. No firm evidence exists showing that the opium poppy was cultivated in Egypt before the Ptolemaic period. Some researchers assume opium was imported from Cyprus and Syria in small jugs whose form resembles the appearance of the poppy.[81] Opium is a milky product derived from the poppy plant (*Papaver somniferum L*) which contains several alkaloids, including morphine, which has a strong sedative effect. The Egyptian expression which has been identified as referring to opium is *špnn nw špn* (Westendorf 1999: 507).[82] If this identification is correct, Egyptian physicians could have used opium as an effective anaesthesia in the treatment of wounds (Sm.41) and abscesses (Sm.46). Also, this material is used in a remedy "to expel the (child's) cry" (Eb.782), and scholars suggest that this remedy must have been truly effective, as in fact opium was still being used extensively for this very purpose in Egypt before its cultivation was outlawed in 1914, as well as in England during the nineteenth century (Merrillees 1962: 292; Nunn 1996: 154–5).[83]

Manniche (1999: 113–4) suggests that the ancient Egyptians would have been well aware of the aromatherapeutic property of the scented oil of acacia leaves. Taking a prescription in the Berlin papyrus which records "A remedy to stop the blood which has been taken to the heart and has spread: dried acacia leaves are ground and mixed with oil or fat. Heat to finger warmth and used as a bandage" (Bln.151), Manniche asserts this could be an excellent example of the Egyptians' understanding of the penetrating quality of aromatic oil that was not inhaled through the nose, but was diffused through pores of the skin and affected the inner hidden parts.

The magico-religious element

Analogy

The homeopathic principle is commonly applied in assumptions of the magical aspect of the Egyptian pharmacology. There are many examples of suggested interpretation such as the sawdust of six different kinds of wood that are employed to cure "weakness of the male member (i.e. impotence)" (Eb.663) through the transmission of the consistency of wood to the penis; the heart of the *mšꜥ*-bird being applied to kill the *pnd*-worm since, the bird is insectivorous in nature, its heart can magically kill the worm (Eb.81); in much the same way, the fat of a *gnw*-bird is to be anointed "to prevent a fly from bitting" (Eb.845), and the *ꜥnꜥrt*-worm, being hairless, was applied "to cause the hair to fall out" (Eb.474) (Ghalioungui 1973: 144). We can also find the pulverized eggshell of an ostrich used to glue a fracture of the skull (Sm.9) (Sigerist 1951: 284) and the ostrich egg for the "clearance of *ꜣdyt*-disease in the eye," based on the great sight of the bird (Eb.409) (Leitz 2005: 54). A very impressive example is the fat of a cat which was placed "to prevent mice from approaching to things" (Eb.847).

Another form of the homeopathic principle is the use of puns.[84] As an example, Gardiner (1915: 265–6) provides an incantation that says "I make a charm for him against thee of *'afai*-plant, which does injury, of onions, which destroy thee, and of honey, which is sweet to men and sour to the dead" (*Zaubersprüche*, recto 2.4).[85] He comments that while the virtues here ascribed to the *'afai*-plant and to honey are of obscure origin, the destructive property attributed to onions is clearly due to the fact that the Egyptian word for onions was *ḥădg* (the vowel is merely guessed), and its phonetic similarity with "to destroy" was *ḥōdg*. Another example Gardiner (1915: 267) presents to us is a material in a prescription of the Ebers papyrus (Eb.733) that reads: "To cure a complaint called 'the working of charms' (*ḥmt-sꜥ*) the following is prescribed: A large beetle (*ḫprr*), whose head and wings have been cut off. To be burnt and put into fat, and then applied." He comments on the word for beetle, being derived from the verb *khōper* (*ḫpr*), "to become," a mutilated beetle would symbolize the frustrated achievement of a purpose; the purpose intended to be frustrated was "the working of

[79] This recognition of the empirical element is what is commonly introduced in articles of Egyptian medicine; see, for instance, Breasted (1930: 59), Sigerist (1951: 340), Leake (1952: 70), Ghalioungui (1973: 143–4), Manniche (1989: 145), Jacob, W. (1993: 38) and Nunn (1996: 144–60). This recognition depends on an identification of the material, and the different assertions for the identification to the material immediately results in the loss of the validity of the identification of the empirical element.

[80] For discussions about opium in ancient Egypt, see Krikorian (1978) and Bisset (1994; 1996); Nunn (1996: 153–6) provides a concise summary.

[81] For details concerning Cypriot base ring juglet, see Merrillees (1962) and Koschel (1996); Reeves (1992: 59) and Nunn (1996: 156) provide a picture of a Cypriot base ring juglet and inverted the seed pod of the opium poppy.

[82] Nunn (1996: 153–6) and Westendorf (1999: 507) are cautious with this identification.

[83] Germer (1979: 328) notes that Opium "zur Zeit als unbekannt angesehen werden muß, eine Beziehung zu Papaver somniferum ist nicht zu belegen," and moreover "gibt es eine größere Anzahl weiterer Pflanzen, die zu diesem Zweck (Beruhigen von Kindern) in der Kinderheilkunde verwendet werden, z. B. Fenchel" (quoted from Westendorf 1992: 215).

[84] Gardiner (1915: 265) states "The very idea of the oral rite is an instance of homoeopathic magic, for language may be said to imitate and image the things which it expresses, and in so far verbal references to a desired effect may have been considered instrumental in producing it." About the use of the pun in Egyptian medicine, see also Dawson's comments (1929: 50–1).

[85] This text is from the Berlin papyrus (3027, B). Dawson (1934: 41) and Sigerist (1951: 283) translate "garlic" instead of Gardiner's "onion."

charms."[86] Miller (1994: 353) explains the hostile property of the *ḏaajs*-plant: "According to one of the dream interpretations in P. Chester Beatty III, no. 7, 9: 'If a man sees himself in a dream, munching *ḏaajs*, (this is) bad—it means hostility.' The alliterative word-play between *ḏaajs* (plant) and hostility (*ḏaajs*), may perhaps suggest that the plant and hostility shared a disagreeable and unpleasant character." Long (1984: 147) notes that the use of the *nỉ3nỉ3*-plant against *nỉ3*-disease in Eb.762 is based on a "sympathie phonétique entre deux termes qui ajoute sa vertu homéopathique à l'efficacité chimique du remède par l'evocation magique des mots."

Another medico-magical principle we can apply to Egyptian pharmacology is the transference of a disease entity into substances that could serve as a medium. There is a treatment for blindness (Eb.356) in which the fluid of a hog's eye and some other substances are made into a remedy and instilled into a patient's ear. Then the following incantation is recited "I have brought this which was applied to the seat of yonder and replace the horrible suffering," and the same principle may have been employed in the treatment of the "pain in one side of the head" (Eb.250) in which the head of a *nʿr*-fish was rubbed on an aching area (Ghalioungui 1973: 18). Here, the use of intuitive analogy in transferring the disease entity is also notable.[87]

Impure ingredients
Materials that are strongly suggestive of their magical property are impure and peculiar materials that are aptly known in German as *Dreckapotheke* (i.e. dirt apothecary). Throughout the Egyptian prescriptions we find extensive use of disagreeable substances including the blood of snake, skin of hippopotamus, dung of crocodile, donkey's hair and teeth, and even excrement of man and urine of a menstruating woman. It is, however, not appropriate to classify of such materials as magical simply because they appear to be weird and curious to us.[88]

Sacerdotal property
The sacerdotal medical property of a substance can be seen to derive from Egyptian religious concepts. Usually the materials acquire their therapeutic property from the reflection of roles played by divinities in Egyptian myths. The case of the association of the "milk of a woman who has born a male child" for burns with the healing practices of the goddess Isis in the myth has already been mentioned (see p. 28). Another example of material with a sacerdotal property is watermelon. In the myth, when the god Seth is pursuing the beautiful goddess Isis, he transforms himself into a bull and scatters his semen on the ground in frustration, and from it grew the watermelon (Manniche 1989: 92). There may be a conceptual connection with the Hieroglyphics for watermelon 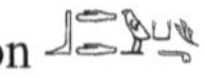 (*bddw-k3*) with this mythological notion because the word can carry the penis determinative 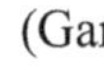 (Gardiner sign-list: D 52). In the Egyptian prescription, the watermelon appears in the treatment (Eb.663) for "weakness of the male member" together with the sawdust of woods, and it can be understood as the application of the sexual property attributed to watermelon. Also, lettuce has a close association with semen in ancient Egypt. This is generally considered to be due to its milky sap, which is reminiscent of semen. Lettuce is associated with the ithyphallic god Min,[89] and in the myth of the contendings of Horus and Seth, Seth became pregnant after eating lettuce on which had been scattered the semen of Horus (Dawson 1932b: 152; Lichtheim 1976: 220; Manniche 1989: 113). Dawson (1932b: 152) asserts that the Egyptians regarded lettuce as an aphrodisiac. One of the uses of lettuce in Egyptian prescriptions is in the remedy "to encourage the growth of hair" (Eb.467), and we may understand that lettuce could stimulate breeding hair just as it could stimulate the genitals. We also find instances where an ibis of wax is placed on charcoal in fumigation treatment "to cause a woman's womb to go to its place" (Eb.795), and this may indicate an association with the god Thoth, the divine patron of physicians, as the ibis was his symbolic form (Herskey 1989: 752).[90]

---

[86] Gardiner also provides another example of the Egyptian use of pun outside pharmacology. One text (Eb.838) mentions "Another to determine the fate of a child on the day he is brought into the world. If he says *ny*, it means he will live; if he says *mbi*, it means he will die." Gardiner (1915: 266) notes that the sound *mbi* resembles the emphatic Egyptian expression for "no," and Halioua *et al.* (2005: 76) comments "No rational explanation has yet been found for this even though we know that *ny* and *mbi* are translated respectively as "yes" and "no."

[87] It is noteworthy that the remedy was applied into the ear for the treatment of the eye; presumably it was believed that the remedy would reach the eye via the *mṯw*; The above descriptions of the homeopathic treatments reveal the variation in the type of analogy applied. There are several ways to classify the type of analogy. For example, Leitz (2005: 44–5) classifies it into 5 categories namely, Isodynamie, Morphoanalogie, Chromoanalogie, Dynamoanalogie and Ergoanalogie, although he notes that such a model of various analogies alone is not sufficient: "Es wird sich im folgenden zeigen, daß es mit einem solchen Modell verschiedener Analogien nicht getan ist; die eigentliche Schwierigkeit besteht in den meisten Fällen vielmehr darin herauszufinden, was genau denn die Analogie ist. In einigen Fällen kommt dabei nichtmedizinischen, vor allem religiösen Texten eine Schlüsselrolle zu; eine andere wichtige Quelle können naturkundliche, insbesondere zoologische Schriften sein" (Leitz 2005: 45).

[88] Dawson (1929: 55–6) states that the use of oil as an ointment is rational, but "the magical element enters when, instead of merely ox-fat, or goose-grease, we find prescriptions introducing the fat of all kinds of different animals, many of them rare and difficult to obtain, such as lion, oryx, hippopotamus, snake, mouse etc" (Eb.465).

[89] Germer (1980: 939) notes "Die Beziehung zwischen dem Fruchtbarkeitsgott Min und dem L. (Lattich) beruht wahrscheinlich auf einer mythischen Verknüpfung des aus der Pflanze bei Anschnitt austretenden Milchsaftes mit der Samenflüssigkeit des Gottes, da der L. auf Grund seiner pharmazeutischen Bestandteile als Aphrodisiakum ungeeignet ist"; See also Germer (2002: 125–8).

[90] Another possible material thought to have sacerdotal healing property is the milk of the donkey. Leitz (2005: 46–7) sees the healing property of the milk of the donkey being derived from its association with the god Seth that the material is used as the "Hauptbestandteil eines Medikaments (pEbers 98) für das Töten der Schmerzstoffe (*wḫdw*). Die unmittelbar folgende Nummer (99) ist ein Alternativerezept mit einer ausführlicheren Überschrift: 'Ein anderes (Heilmittel) für das Töten der Schmerzstoffe und das Beseitigen des Giftsamens (*ʿ3ʿ*) eines Toten oder einer Toten im Bauch eines Mannes oder einer Frau.' Über diesen Giftsamen und dessed Verbreitung durch den eselsgestaltigen Gott Seth ist man seit den Forschungen WESTENDORFs über altägyptische Incubusvorstellungen gut unterrichtet … Der Spruch 26 des Londoner medizinischen Papyrus, der sich gegen den Giftsamen richtet, soll über einem steifen Phallus eines Esels aus Gebäck gesprochen werden, der danach einer Katze zum Fressen vorgeworfen wird. Die Verbindungen des Gottes Seth, des potentiellen Incubus,

Duplication of interpretations

Occasionally, an overlap of interpretations based on empirico-rational and magico-religious principles occurs. Honey, for instance, is the most frequently used material throughout the prescriptions, and most treatments of injury employ honey. Honey is, in fact, a highly effective antiseptic, mainly due to its hypertonic property that can kill micro-organisms along an osmotic gradient (i.e. by drawing water out of them) and also due to its gluconic acid and hydrogen peroxide which are mildly antibacterial (Majno 1975: 117–18; Estes 1989: 69; Houten 1980: 101).[91] But in one incantation (Berlin Papyrus 3027, B) we can infer honey's magical force to expel demonical disease from the statement "I have made for him (the patient) a protective charm against you (the demonical entity) consisting of evil smelling herbs, of garlic which is harmful to you, and of honey which is sweet for the living but horrible to the dead" (Dawson 1934: 41; Sigerist 1951: 283). In a similar fashion, fresh meat, which is almost always applied in the Edwin Smith papyrus to wounds on the first day, is a rational hemostatic because meat can act as a cushion and stop haemorrhaging by means of pressure (Sigerist 1951: 344; Ghalioungui 1973: 144).[92] But it is also possible to assume the presence of a homeopathic principle, "flesh mends flesh" (Estes 1989: 64). Similarly, the sycamore fig, being high in ficin content, produces a mild laxative effect and is found being used for this purpose (e.g. Eb.39) (Weeks 1995: 1796), but the strong association of the sycamore and the goddess Isis and Hathor is frequently showed in Egyptian mythology, and thus the sycamore may have been attributed divine curative power in ancient Egypt.

Duplication of interpretation can occur even with weird materials. One text in the Book of the Dead (Spell 53) illustrates that one of the fears of the deceased was to lack food or drink and to be compelled to eat his own excreta expressed as "I detest what is detestable, I will not eat faeces, I will not drink urine" (Faulkner 1972: 65). This concept accords well with the medical incantation in the Hearst papyrus (He.85b) which recites "flow out of my body, I have brought you (the evil spirit) excrement to eat." Thus we may consider that a force to expel the dead who brought disease was attributed to excreta. Pinch (1994: 134) regards this in a different way, suggesting the use of excrement may have been motivated by the homeopathic principle: since many diseases arise from faecal residue and *wḫdw* in the belly, application of excreta has been used to encourage the residue to come down. Contrary to these interpretations, some scholars argue for a rational medicinal use of excreta. It is known that certain substances produced by micro-organisms living in human and animal bodies possess an antimicrobial action of their own, and this can be excreted through faeces and urine, and thus excreta can contain effective antibiotics (Reeves 1992: 59–60; Stetter 1933: 155). Other scholars emphasise the ammoniacal properties of excreta that produce an antiseptic effect when applied to wounds (Breasted 1930: 59; Pinch 1994: 134). Early in the twentieth century, Maspéro (1909: 269) also pointed out the efficacy of ammonia in excreta: "it is certainly less disagreeable to apply ammonia, or medicament made with ammonia, where the Egyptians prescribe urine, or the excrements of certain animals, but the results were the same, and the ammonia imprisoned in those repugnant substances acted in exactly the same manner as if it had been chemically prepared; it may be that, mingled with organic substances, its action was less harsh than it is in the case of pure ammonia of our laboratories."

This approach, which includes empirico-rational and magico-religious perspectives, is convincing to a degree. The bactericidal power of malachite and some other materials demonstrated by Majno (1975: 112–15) is convincing, and the Egyptian use of malachite to draw out inflammation from the "mouth of a wound" (Sm.46) and for burns (Eb.491) shows rationality.[93] But the use of malachite in the prescription "to make that flesh grow" (Eb.533) may be due to the green colour of malachite, which is the same colour as plants, suggesting a property of growing. There are in fact a great many more duplications in interpretation which can be enumerated. This is due to the fact that many substances actually exhibit their therapeutic efficacy, as, for instance, the antiseptic quality in onion, garlic, leek, cinnamon, beer, frankincense, myrrh, storax, benzoni, turpentine, sagapen, manna, laudanum, acacia and also minerals like copper and malachite are affirmed for quite different reasons (Leake 1952: 70; Manniche 1989: 89; Pahor 1992: 681; Reeves 1992: 60; Sigerist 1951: 340; Stetter 1993: 115).[94] Also, the different animal products such as fat, milk, honey and wax can show a demulcent and sedative effect (Ghalioungui 1973: 144).

Interpreting the religious virtue of substances may be easier than unravelling the conventions of rationality because Egyptian religion commonly makes associations between substances, especially of plants, and deities. In a magical text (British Museum papyrus No. 10051, Salt 825), for instance, a tear from the god Horus turns into gum anti (i.e. "myrrh"); a tear from the god Ra becomes "flies that build" (i.e. "bees") that produce honey and wax; blood from the nose of the god Geb turns into a cedar tree; blood of the gods Osiris and Seth becomes a Nart tree and sweat of the goddess Isis and Nephthys turns into plants (Budge 1928: 24; Dawson 1929: 10). Barley is a symbol of the resurrection of the god Osiris and was grown in a

zum Esel sind weit verbreitet; der Esel war … in der ägyptischen Schrift normalerweise mit einem Phallus determiniert … Da der Giftsame und die als vergleichbar angesehenen Schmerzstoffe auf den eselsgestaltigen Seth zurückgehen können, versucht man in einem von mehreren Rezepten, dies Leiden durch die Verwendung von Eselsmilch zu heilen."

[91] Bergman (1983: 374) notes that the application of honey for wound healing was used by Russian soldiers in World War I.

[92] Breasted (1930: 97) notes that meat is still used as a folk medicine in this way up to the present.

[93] For a detailed description of the chemotherapeutic principle of copper, see Weser (1987).

[94] General antiseptic property of plants is due to their secondary metabolites, see p. 19.

rough wooden frame in the form of Osiris that is known as an "Osiris bed."[95] Even simple water can be assumed to have an association with deities for it is the symbol of the Nile-god Hapi who provides life and also of the great watery abyss (*nun*) from which the first god Ra or Khepri sprang.

The overlap in interpretations need not constitute a problem. Firstly, the interpretations are all hypothetical and secondly, in antiquity, the rational aspect and religious concepts are not perceived as incompatible due to the integrity of science and religion. Nevertheless, modern-day understanding through the application of two contradictory perspectives can often lead to a loss of focus. We should, therefore, be aware that although the empirico-rational and magico-religious elements are both useful criteria for us, they do not necessarily accurately reflect the thoughts of ancient Egyptians.

Rendering the meaning of materials

A further difficulty appears, when considering the Egyptian materia medica, in assuming a literal translation of medicinal materials. It is very common in many cultures for materials, particularly plants, to be referred to by slang terms or nicknames. In English, for example, "goosefoot" refers to *Chenopodium anthelminticum*, "fox gloves" is *digitalis* and "ladies" means *belladonna*[96]; in Arabic *abu en noum* (lit. "father's sleep") designates the poppy's flower (Ghalioungui 1973: 141; Manniche 1989: 130). In Japanese *taka no tsume* (lit. "claw of hawk") denotes cayenne. Also, in antiquity, in Coptic ⲗⲁⲥ ⲛⲉⲓⲟⲙ (lit. "tongue of the sea") meant the back part of an octopus or cuttlebone (Sobhy 1938: 14; Stetter 1993: 43; Westendorf 1999: 501). Ghaliougui (1973: 140–1) introduces interesting parallels between the ancient Egyptian and Arabic word whereby the *ḥs n ꜥff* (lit. "fly's dirt") (e.g. Eb.782) in the Egyptian text is compared with *nesheshet el debban* (lit. "fly's dirt"), the modern popular name of *Silena rubellis* in Arabic; and the strange substance called *ḫfꜥ-ꜥi-ꜣm-ꜥi* (lit. "my hand holds, my hand grasps") that carries the plant determinative in the Egyptian prescription (Eb.166) is compared with *qef wanzor* (lit. "stop and look"), corrupted into *qafandar*, which denotes *Ruscus alexandrinus*. Tait (1991: 47, 60, 74) notes that words such as *iny-pꜣ-nty-rt* (lit. "the stone which grows"), *sꜣt-pꜣ-nty-sḏr* (lit. "Daughter of the one who is asleep") and *bn-iw-pꜣ-gm-rn.i* (lit. "There is no finding my name") appear as a name of a herb in the demotic papyrus (Carlsberg 230). Sobhy (1938: 14) compares Coptic *las en jom* with Egyptian *ns-š* (lit. "tongue of pond") and tentatively equates it with cuttlebone.

Another aspect to consider is the jargon of physicians. A Greco-Egyptian magical papyrus named "interpretations" (PGM XII.401–44) lists the secret meaning of ingredients. It mentions renderings like "snake's head" meaning a "leech", "crocodile dung" meaning "Ethiopian soil", "hair of Hamadryas baboon" meaning "dill seed", "man's bile" meaning "turnip sap", "blood of geese" meaning a "mulberry tree's milk" and "semen of Ammon" meaning "houseleek," etc. (Betz 1986: 167–9). It is difficult to say whether these name substitutions dating to the Greek period can also be applied to earlier Egyptian medical texts. With regard to this text, Pinch (1994: 80) comments that such substitutions as "crocodile dung" for "Ethiopian soil" may probably be a late rationalization of ingredients rather than a true explanation for all periods.[97]

The rendering of meaning reminds us of the word "secret," which occasionally appears in Egyptian papyri including the "Beginning of the Physician's Secret" (Eb.854a = Sm.1 Gloss A), "secret herbal remedy which is made by the physician" (Eb.188) or ""you shall prepare for him the secret remedy" (Eb.206) (see p. 61-2). Thus the Egyptian terms for their materia medica may have been jargon or secret appellations of the physicians, concealing their secret specialist knowledge of pharmacology. Indeed some scholars suggest several Egyptian material terms to be metaphors or figurative names. It has been suggested, for instance, that material from a donkey such as "ear of donkey" (Eb.770), "head of donkey" (Eb.106), "leg of donkey" (Eb.108) and "tooth of donkey' (Eb.470) are kinds of plants (Ghalioungui 1987: 35, 131, 197; Grapow 1958: 67, 189). Also, the term *sd-pnw* (lit. "mouse tail") (Eb.160), which carries the plant determinative, or terms which are not represent materials like *šwt-ḏḥwti* (lit. "Thot's feather")[98] (Eb. 299, 669) and *irt-pt* (lit. "heaven's eye") (Eb.776) may be safely understood to be mere herbs (Ghalioungui 1973: 140). Bardinet (1999) concludes that *ḥs n ꜥff* (lit. "fly's dirt") is an expression designating a propolis. Ghalioungui (1973: 141) comments: "One could fancy a *swnw*'s amusement if he heard us seriously state that he made ointments with the head or leg of a donkey (Eb.160, 108), dissolved donkey's (sic. pig's) teeth in a watery mixture (Eb.316), or dressed a wound with pig's teeth (Eb.580). We would certainly be as abashed if we found historians in 4000 A.D. wondering at the use of fox gloves (*digitalis*) or powder of handsome ladies (*belladonna*)." [99]

[95] Also called a "Corn-mummy." In the Osirian Festival of Khoiak the mould in the shape of the Osiris-figure with sprouting seeds, which imply life after death, was placed in a trough called *ḥspt* ("garden") (Griffiths 1982: 630).

[96] Mann (2000: 22) notes "Juice from belladonna berries when squeezed into the eyes produces dilation of the pupils, and was thus much used by Renaissance ladies to impart a 'doe-eyed beauty' look—hence the name 'belladonna' (Italian for 'beautiful woman')."

[97] The Egyptian term commonly translated as "dung of crocodile" is *tꜣ-msḥ*, which literary means "earth of crocodile" (Westendorf 1999: 494).

[98] Westendorf (1999: 506) reads the term *šw.t-Nmtj* ("Feder des Nemti"); The reading is based on the identification with the Greek πτερου ίβες "Kriechendes Fünffinger-Kraut," and he notes "Aber vielleicht hat in der Spätzeit bei gewissen Schreibungen eine Verwechslung des unbekannten Gottes Nemti mit dem bedeutenderen Thot stattgefunden wie bei den Ägyptologen" (Westendorf 1999: 506–7).

[99] Ghalioungui (1961: 17) notes that descriptive names or cryptograms were used by alchemists in the Middle Ages to keep their manipulations secret.

CHAPTER 4

Indication of Presence of Theories in Egyptian Medicine

The Egyptian medical texts are essentially practical by nature, dealing with individual factual cases rather than providing systematic explanatory teachings of medicine. Reymond (1984: 186) notes that the study of the Egyptian medicine presents us with rather curious and contrasting aspects: (a) the theoretical knowledge of medical matters, which is largely undocumented and (b) the practical expression of that knowledge in the contents of papyri. Assumptions of the presence of an elaborate medical theory in Egyptian medicine, which goes beyond simple empirical medicine and primitive mytho-magical healing, have been made, and actually a close study of Egyptian medicine reveals that such assumption is not too speculative but significant to make a consideration upon it.

Following the publications of the medical papyri, it was not long before scholars of Egyptian medicine realized the significance and value of comparative studies, particularly with Greek medicine, for a consideration of the elaborated Egyptian medical theory because these publications revealed many signs of influence from Egyptian to Greek medicine as well as medicines of later periods, and this could lead to an assumption that the medical theory, which was considered to be particular to the Greek medicine, was originated in ancient Egypt and was transmitted into Greek medicine. This, in turn, indicates the Egyptians' achievement of formulating a specific medical theory.

4.1 Egyptian influence on Greek and later medicines

The high reputation of Egyptian physicians and their medicine in antiquity is well attested to in various records. Homer's Odyssey (950BC; IV, 227–32) mentions Egypt as a land "which produces drugs in abundance, a great many mixtures of which are salutary and a great many others are baneful; and there every man is a physician, wise above humankind, for they are race of Paeëon" (based on trans. Murray 1995: 135). Herodotus (III, 129) mentions that Darius was accustomed "to keep in attendance certain Egyptian doctors, who had a reputation for the highest eminence in their profession" (trans. Sélincourt 1996: 204). Several letters from rulers of neighbouring countries demanding Egyptian medical treatment indicates the high value accorded to Egyptian medicine in antiquity.[100] Judging from the evidence in medical writings, it seems there was no influence between Egypt and Mesopotamia, and that these cultures were relatively independent during the Dynastic period.[101] But the Hittite records show a degree of local adoption of Egyptian medicine probably through a steady importation of Egyptian physicians and remedies to the Anatolian court (Ritner 2001b: 355). As for Greek medicine, much evidence of strong Egyptian influence has been found.

Egyptian influence on Greek medicine

The Kahun (Kh.19–27), Berlin (Bln.193–9) and Carlsberg papyri contain an extraordinary series of tests for fertility, pregnancy and methods for determining the sex of an unborn child. The Kahun papyrus, which is hitherto the oldest discovered medical papyrus (1800 BC), contains a test for fertility (Kh.28), and a parallel test (Car.IV, 1, x+4–6) can be found in the Carlsberg papyrus of a later period (1300 BC). The text reads "(to determine) who will (bear children) and who will not, you should then cause the bulb of an onion to spend the night in her flesh (*iwf*: i.e. vagina) until dawn. If the odour appears in her mouth, she will bear (children). If (it does not), she will never (bear children)."[102] We can find this text in a modified

[100] Ghalioungui (1983: 76–80) introduces several letters from kings of Ugarit and the Hittites to pharaohs demanding an Egyptian physician; About the letters from the Hittites, see also Edel (1976: 125–8); For the reputation of Egyptian physician, see Nunn (1996: 131–2).

[101] In later Hellenistic and Roman times, however, there is evidence for Babylonian astrology on Egyptian medicine.

[102] In this work, the translations from the Kahun papyrus are chiefly based on Stevens' (1975) translation; Stephan (2005: 94) recognises here an Egyptian anatomical principle: "Die Geschlechtsorgane der Frau sind offenbar als durchgehender vertikaler Kanal gedacht, vergleichbar etwa dem Verdauungskanal," and he notes that "Überhaupt ist Paradigma von Kanälen, die den Körper durchziehen, abgeleitet vom Bewässerungssystem der Felder, eine prägende Vorstellung der ägyptischen Physiologie, zuerst von Westendorf beschrieben, und seither unter dem Namen 'Nilstromtheorie' bekannt" (Stephan 2005:

form in the Hippocratic corpus (*On Sterility*, *Aphorism* V, 59; *On Diseases of Women* VIII, 416) (Saunders 1963: 117–18; Nunn 1996: 192; Stephan 2005: 94). A pregnancy prognostication method is described in the texts of the Kahun (Kh.26) and Berlin (Bln.193) papyri and is entitled "To recognise who will be pregnant and who will not be pregnant":

> She lies down (while) you smear her breast and her arms and her two shoulders with new oil. You rise early in the morning to examine her. (If) you find her *mṯw* fresh and good, none being sunken, bearing children will be *ḥtp* (i.e. satisfactory). (If) you find them sunken like the skin of her limbs, this means *bnd* (difficulty?). If you find them green and dark at the time of examining them, she will bear children late.

Ghalioungui (1973: 112) comments on this passage: "Allowing for difficulties in interpreting these archaic texts, it is a fact that in pregnancy the skin is characteristically pigmented (chloasma) and the breasts are heavy and congested."[103] We find that the Hippocratic corpus (*Aphorism* V, 37) also refers to the consistency of the breasts as a sign of pregnancy.

The Berlin papyrus (Bln.198) also provides another test by checking the eyes of a woman stating that "if the one (eye) is like that of an Asiatic, the other like that of a negress, then she will not bear (while) if you find colour in one of them, then she will bear." The same method is introduced in the Carlsberg papyrus (Car.VI 2, 1–3) and utilized by Hippocrates (*On Sterile Women* III, 215) (Ghalioungui 1968: 101).[104] An alternative method which is also contained in the Berlin papyrus (Bln.193, 194) employs *bddw-k3* (watermelon) together with the "milk of a woman who has born a male child," which should be administered to the vagina or rubbed onto the woman's back. This will cause vomiting if she can conceive, but she will merely suffer from indigestion if she has not. The identical text exists in the Hippocratic corpus (*On Sterile* VI) (Dawson 1927: 297–8; Ghalioungui 1960: 299).[105]

Some surgical practices recorded in the Edwin Smith papyrus are also found in the Greek medical texts. The operation for the treatment of a dislocated mandible by Egyptians (Sm.25) is almost identical to the method practiced by Hippocratic physicians (*On Joints*, XXX-XXXI) (Ghalioungui 1969b: 165), and there is an essential similarity in the conception of the three basic types of injury between in the Edwin Smith papyrus and the Hippocratic texts (*On Wounds in the Head*) (Iversen 1953: 168–9) (see p. 59). A striking fact is that the text concerning the fracture of the clavicle (Sm.35) and the fracture of the nose (Sm.11) appear in the same wording and format in the Hippocratic texts of *Peri Arthrôn* (*On Joints* XIV-XV, XXXVII-XXVIII) (Ghalioungui 1960: 298–9; 1968: 99; 1973: 42). These observations are evidence of direct translation of the Egyptian medical texts into the Greek language. Moreover, many prescriptions of the Ebers papyrus can be found in the Greek medical texts (e.g. Eb.101, 193b, 201b, 565 and 594 in the works of Dioscorides I, iv), and they again appear almost word for word, and similar prescriptions occur even in Byzantine texts (e.g. *Codex Paulinae Lipsiensis*) (Saunders 1963: 15; Ghalioungui 1973: 114; Stevens 1975: 952). In fact we can find ample evidence which indicates direct transmission of Egyptian medicine into Greek and later medicines.

As in the medicine of the Egyptians and in many other medicines, the Greek prescriptions employ many herbs and other ordinary medicinal substances, but there are materials that may indicate the influence of Egypt on the Greek materia medica. Evidence of this is seen in the substances specifically termed "Egyptian" including "white Egyptian oil", "Egyptian salt", "Egyptian saffron," and the "*bolbion* seen especially in Egyptian grain fields" (e.g. Hippocratic corpus, *On Women's Diseases* 1.37, 75, 78; 2.181) and materials of Egyptian origin such as "red natron" and of Egyptian culture such as "milk of a woman who has born a male child" (e.g. Hippocratic corpus, *Sterile Women* 8.214, *De morbis Mulierum* 1.20; Dioscorides, *De Materia Medica* 5.99; Pliny, *Historia Naturalis* 20.51, 134) (Dawson 1932a: 12–13; Ghalioungui 1960: 296–7; Prioreschi 2003: 156).[106] Often one can identify Greek names for medicinal substances as being Egyptian borrowings including Egyptian *hbny* (ebony) and Greek *ebenon*, *ḳmyt* (gum) and *kómmi*, *msdmt* (antimony) and *stimmi*,[107] and *gsfn* and *sagapinon*[108] (Ghalioungui 1960: 297; 1986: 9–16; Marganne 1993: 37–8).[109] Ghalioungui (1968: 98–9) notices some possible associations between Egyptian and Greek medicinal substances, and in one case he mentions "… A similar double affiliation in both name and indication is found in the use of petroleum for different eye diseases (Eb.380, 412; Dioscorides I, 73). It is interesting that "petroleum" which is derived from *petra*, a rock, and *oleum*, oil, is the exact counterpart of its Egyptian name, *mrḥt ḫ3st* or "that which comes from the desert" (Eb.76), the word desert being practically synonymous with stone or rock (Ghalioungui 1968: 99).[110]

94).

[103] Nunn (1996: 192) also notes: "Dilated veins over the breasts are well known as an early sign of pregnancy."

[104] Ghalioungui (1973: 112) also points out: "Hippocrates foretold the infant's sex by the colour of the mother's eyes (Aph. 5, XLII)."

[105] In this Hippocratic text, the term *boutiron* is identified by Dawson with watermelon, in Egyptian *bddw*. But Ghalioungui (1973: 114) comments "Philologists are better qualified to decide whether these two words are close enough, in spite of the dissimilarity of the last consonant, to justify this identification."

[106] Ghalioungui (1960: 297) states that the material is purely Egyptian origin and notes "le lait de femme était considéré comme nocif par certains peoples d'Orient, comme le Assyro-Babyloniens."

[107] Breasted (1930: 489) notes that *msdmt* has been corrupted into Coptic ⲥⲧⲏⲙ, Greek στίμμι and finally Latin *stibium*.

[108] Greek σαγαπηνον = gsfn > sgfn > sgpn ? (Westendorf 1999: 509).

[109] In Greek pharmacopeia, there are many examples of the borrowing of the Egyptian term including *sry* and *nṯry*. For more hypothetical assertions of possible signs of Egyptian influence on Greek, see Ghalioungui (1989) and Marganne (1993); concerning the identification of the *k3k3*-plant as the castor-oil plant and its relationship with *kiki*, see Dawson (1929) and also Westendorf (1999: 508).

[110] Ghalioungui (1960: 298–9) also notes some possible association between Egyptian and Greek anatomo-physiological terms. An

In striking contrast to the Greeks' frequent reference to Egyptian medicine, there is no evidence suggesting direct translation of Mesopotamian medical texts into Greek medical writings. But undoubtedly there were significant influences from Mesopotamian medicine on Greek medicine because, similar to the influence of Egyptian materia medica, there are a number of Greek words that are mere transliterations of the Assyrian.[111]

Egyptian influence on later medicines

The local continuation of pharaonic medical practices in later periods is well attested to in the texts of Coptic medicine, which is often considered to be the direct successor of Egyptian medicine. Just as the Greek medical texts use ἄλλως or ἄλλο in reference to an alternative prescription, showing the Greek adoption of the ancient Egyptian textual format "another" or "another remedy," the Coptic medical texts also follow this style of format (Breasted 1930: 477).

The extant texts of the Crocodilopolis medical papyrus (P.Vindib, D 6257), which are written in Demotic, are dated to around the second century AD, but the original is thought to belong to the early Ptolemaic Period; and occasionally scholars even notice features of Middle Egyptian, indicating that some of the texts are copies of much older medical texts.[112] It has also been recognised, however, that the addition of the newer elements, which include about 60 plants and 5 minerals used in the Crocodilopolis papyrus, are not attested in pharaonic texts, and they are presumed to have come to Egypt during the Late and Ptolemaic Period (Nunn 1996: 208; Ritner 2000: 113). It is noteworthy that the ratio of the emergence of newer material is relatively high, since only 201 medicinal materials are used in this papyrus.

The medicine of the early Coptic period is actually little understood, mainly due to scarcity of evidence. But the continuing uses of the ancient materia medica such as red natron and "milk of a woman who has born a male child" found throughout the Coptic medical papyri is noticeable. Among several Coptic medical papyri, the Chassinat papyrus of the 9th–10th century AD is a good source as it provides us with clearer views of Coptic medicine.[113] The significant feature showed by the Chassinat papyrus is its inclusion of numerous Greek and Arabic words. The names of some medicinal materials are Greek and Arabic written in the Coptic alphabet with the same pronunciation. Gammal (1989: 727–30) notes that the author of the Chassinat papyrus was proficient in both Coptic and Arabic by pointing to Arabic names like *tutia*, *helteet*, *kalkh* and *malh andarani* as well as specific pharmaceutical preparations like *el-bouroud* (i.e. dried powder used for eye infection) and *saout* (snuffs) used properly. Gammal (1989: 730) comments on the Arabic influence on Coptic medicine: "Coptic and Greek medicine were very similar to each other during the first few centuries of Christianity, but differs to a great extent especially after the Arab-Islamic invasion of Egypt in 641 AD, during which the new religion affected enormously many of the cultural and scientific aspects of the Egyptian, although Greek influence was still apparent, but to a lesser extent."

There are, in fact, many more indications of Egyptian influence found in the Greek, Roman, Coptic, Arabic and even Persian, Syriac and Hebrew medicine. The Egyptian influence on Hebrew medicine, for instance, is seen in the Pentateuch[114] in which many names of diseases and few terminological expressions are coined after Egyptian patterns. Yahuda (1947: 564) assumes that a Hebrew word *gabbachat* (Leviticus 13, 42–3), which is traditionally interpreted as "baldness of the forehead," is from the Egyptian *gmḥt* ("temples") (Eb.854c), and he compares Hebrew *qubbã* (Numbers 25, 8), which is generally interpreted as "belly" or "genitals," with Egyptian *ḳꜣbt* ("breast") (Sm.XI, 23) (Yahuda 1947: 565). Also, Yahuda (1947: 559–60) notes that the Hebrew term *shechin*, which appears to refere to several sorts of skin disease, is mentioned in the Pentateuch among other diseases expressly characterised as "Egyptian ills" (Leviticus 13, 18), or the skin disease is refered to as "*shechin* of Egypt" (Deuteronomy 28, 27), and he compares this term with Egyptian *sẖn* which describes a swelling (Erman 1953: 254).[115] Also, in the case of the Hebrew word *abábúoth*, which means "blains like blossoms," he states that a Egyptian text on an enlarged gland which is "like *pꜥpꜥyt* " (Eb.857) can be understood as "blains which break out like blossoms" (Yahuda 1947: 560).[116]

The evidence of Greek and Arabic influences on Coptic medicine are all clear indications of the complex interchange, interaction and interfusion of medicine among cultures which occurred in the course of medical history. A great continuity in the practice of medicine is also evident at the same time as we find that the Chassinat

example is the Egyptian term for the stomach *r n ib* (lit. "mouth of the heart"), which is compared with Greek *stomachos* that is derived from *atoma*, the mouth.

[111] Some examples of cases are provided by Horgan (1949: 34).

[112] For a detailed study of the Crocodilopolis papyrus, see Reymond (1976).

[113] For a detailed study of Chassinat papyrus, see Chassinat (1921) and also Westendorf (1999: 539–40).

[114] This refers to the Hebrew Bible's books of *Bereshit* (Genesis), *Shemot* (Exodus), *Vayiqra* (Leviticus), *Bemidbar* (Numbers) and *Debarim* (Deuteronomy) (Edghill 1963: 744–8).

[115] This term occurs in two places in the Ebers papyrus (Eb.193, 207) but not as a skin disease.

[116] Yahuda (1947) suggests many other possible associations between Hebrew and Egyptian medical terms. Yahuda (1947: 550) states that the philological study reveals the extent of the influence of Egyptian medicine in early times (15th century BC) on the Hebrews, and he also notes "it is possible that either of these parallels may be accidental or explained from the common nature of the disease, and hence derived from a different word of similar meaning. But the cumulative evidence in form and meaning of the many instances quoted is a sufficient indication of a common linguistic basis for their derivation" (Yahuda 1947: 559); Halioua *et al.* (2005: 186) notes "a remedy for a disease of the eyes mentioned in one of the apocryphal books of the Bible, the Book of Tobit (6: 4–12)—an ointment of bile—is strikingly like ones found in the Ebers papyrus (Ebers.347, 360)."

papyrus contains some textual copies of the earlier Zwega Coptic papyrus of the 7th–8th century, but some texts of the Chassinat papyrus appear later in the Arabic works of Ibn Sina (Avicenna) (Gammal 1989: 729–30).

The texts for treatment of fractures of the clavicle and nose in the Edwin Smith papyrus, which were translated into Greek in the Hippocratic corpus, also appear again word for word in the Arabic text of Ibn Sina (Ghalioungui 1967b: 851). The Egyptian use of menstrual blood—"let her menstruation come in its beginning, and her belly and thighs are rubbed therewith, her breast does not fall" (Eb.808)—is comparable with an Arabic test of the 8th century: "if you wish to keep a girl's breast upright, not falling down, take her menstrual blood at the beginning of her period and anoint her nipple therewith; they will not fall, and will remain upright. This is a marvellous and tried secret" (*Al-Demiry* I, 51) (Ghalioungui 1969a: 43). The great continuity of medicine is showed in the persistence and spread of Egyptian medicine into Medieval Europe and even into the present period as Ghalioungui (1966b: 65–8; 1977: 145) notices similar practices are current among the Beduin of the Sinai Peninsula.

One striking example is the Egyptian method "to determine the sex of an unborn child" (Bln.199; Car.III, 1). It recommends that the woman moisten the seed of emmer (*bdt*) and barley (*it*) with her urine every day, and if they both grow, she will bear. If barley grows, it means a male child; if the emmer grows, it means a female; if neither grow, she will not bear,[117] and this particular method is mentioned by Galen (*De Remedies Parabilibus* 2, 26) and also in a German book written by Peter Boyer in the seventeenth century as well as in a German book by Paulini (1734) and in English books of the following century called "The Experienced Midwife" or "The Birth of Mankind" (Dawson 1927: 296–302; Erman 1894, reprinted in 1969: 364; Prioreschi 2003: 154; Stephan 2005: 95).[118] Also, the test for a woman's ability to conceive by use of the onion (see p. 41) is mentioned in an eighteenth century German work by Nicolai Venette (*Von der Erzeugung des Menschen*) (1711) (Stephan 2005: 94). Moreover, the test for determining the sex of unborn child by use of barley and emmer as well as the test for a woman's ability to conceive by onion pessary are mentioned in an Arabic text (*Al-Demiry*) (Ghalioungui 1969a: 43) and have been reported as being practiced in Anatolia in the 1960s (Ghalioungui 1968: 101; Harris 1971: 123). Also, the material "mylke of a woman that berythe a knaue child" appears in English medical compositions of the fourteenth century as well as in German *Arzneibücher* (Dawson 1932a: 12–5; Harris 1971: 117).

From this we can reasonably assume that Egyptian medicine was handed down probably from Alexandria as a gateway to Greece and then transmitted to Rome, the Arab world and then Europe mainly through copying and translating the texts and perhaps partially through oral transmission. Saunders (1963: 16–17) provides a description of a fragmentary view of the course of transmission:

> Intermediate sources appear to have been in many instances the writings of Byzantine physicians, who in turn were dependent upon still earlier Greek sources. An important example is the Byzantine physician Muscio (*fl. c.* 500 A.D.), whose text is largely derived from the *gynecology* of Soranus (*fl. c.* 100 A.D.), but with additions from many others. It passed under the erroneous name of Moschion to become the most influential of writings on diseases of women during the Renaissance. The famous "Rosengarten" of Eucharius Rösslin, first published in 1513 and thereafter translated with various additions into French, English, Dutch, and Spanish, was heavily indebted to the so-called Moschion, and was doubtless the medium which gave wide currency in the popular medical writings of Europe to these Ancient Egyptian beliefs on gynecology from nearly five thousand years earlier—surely one of the most ancient of survivals in literature.

So far, no intermediary medical writings have been discovered that can fill in the gap of more than 1000 years from the time of the surviving ancient Egyptian medical papyri to the time of the Greek medical texts in which many Egyptian borrowings are incorporated. But certainly, just as in Saunder's description of the transmission, many medical texts must have been produced through copying activities. Saunder's description also points to the fact that the different medicines can be gathered and mixed into newer works of medicine, often undergoing additions and modifications over time. Another important factor in the process is the fact that the medical writings of an authoritative physician of a period can appear as the most influential and authoritative medical work to a later period and yet his writings were produced on the basis of earlier medical works.[119]

We can also find signs of the preservation of ancient Egyptian medicine in the form of folk medicine in Egypt today. But folk medicine, unlike transmission in writing, lacks evidence in tangible form for chronological development, and the persistence of ancient Egyptian medicine into it is

[117] Generally the principle of this method is understood as being based on the association of the gender of the cereals in a linguistic sense with the sex of the unborn child, but there does not seem to be general agreement among Egyptologists on the rendering of the Egyptian names of cereals. Ghalioungui (1963: 241) notes that Wreszinski and Dawson translate them by wheat for boys and spelt for girls, whereas Iversen gives wheat and barley; and Grapow translates them by barley for boys and emmer for girls; Westendorf (1999: 526) notes that the principle of analogy (i.e. linguistic gender and sex) used here is "die Analogie der Wort-Magie … in der zur Geschlechtsbestimmung des Kindes das unterschiedliche Genus von *jtj* 'Gerste' und *bd.t* 'Emmer' dient."

[118] Scholars have noted that the cereals in the German mediaeval version are reversed probably due to the opposite linguistic gender of the words in German (Harris 1971: 124; Ghalioungui 1973: 113).

[119] Today the plant medicines are sometimes called Galenical, from the well-known Roman physician Galen, to distinguish them from modern synthesized drugs; but we should be aware that the medicine of Galen is, in turn, based largely on Hippocratic medicine.

difficult to assert. The following are suggested examples for this. The use of the blood of a bat and lizard as a means of hindering the growth of hair is still popular practice among Egyptian peasants, though lizard's blood has been replaced by frog's blood (Dawson 1925: 221–7; Meyerhof 1940: 306; Säve-Söderbergh 1961: 267). The ancient Egyptian prescription against *ḥmwt s3w*-disease (Eb.733) recommends "a big beetle; cut off his head and his wings, boil him, put him in oil and lay him out. Then cook his head and his wings, put them in snake fat, boil and let the patient drink the mixture"; and this same recipe, except for snake fat being replaced by ordinary oil, is used in modern folk medicine to cure haemorrhoids (Erman 1894, reprinted in 1969: 363; Ghalioungui 1969a: 42; Stetter 1993: 103–4). Dawson (1924: 83–6) notices the similar use of a mouse for a child's medicine. Sobhy (1938; 1950; 1952) also notes many signs of the preservation of ancient medicine in modern folk medicine, and he emphasises some of the ancient Egyptian medical terms which have persisted into present Egyptian Arabic. One impressive example that he provides is that of the pomegranate which is used in an ancient Egyptian prescription for killing worms of the abdomen, and the potency of this material against ascaris is now well-known (Sobhy 1952: 626–8). A decoction of the roots of pomegranate is used domestically for the treatment of ascaris even today, particularly in Upper Egypt. Sobhy mentions how interesting it is that throughout Egypt, modern Egyptians call ascaris the "serpent of the abdomen" in Arabic as the ancient Egyptian words for worms carry the snake determinative, and in one case the word has the same phonetic value as word for the snake. In his study he asserts that the comparative study of local Egyptian-Arabic disease names which seem to be related to ancient disease names from the medical papyri may lead to the identification of the diseases of the ancient medical papyri.[120]

4.2 Egyptian and Greek medical theories

We have noted a great deal of evidence for a strong influence of Egyptian medicine on Greek medicine as well as on the medicines of various cultures of later periods. A pertinent question in this regard concerns the extent of Egyptian medical influence that it is reasonable to assume. There are only a limited number of fragments of ancient Egyptian medical writing available to us, but we can still ascertain a number of instances where evidence of Egyptian medicine that has been transmitted into Greek and other medicines can be discerned. One would speculate that the Greek medical texts regarded as originating in Greece may in fact have been mere translations of Egyptian texts that have since been lost, or one would postulate that the Greek medical writings may have been based on what the Greeks learnt from Egypt. Two opposing opinions have been voiced since the early stage of the study of medicine in antiquity. One asserts that the Greeks received little from Egyptian medicine and that therefore there is little Egyptian influence in the formulation of Greek medicine (e.g. Staden and Frase; see p. 48-9). The other interpretation insists that Greek medicine owed much to Egyptian medicine (e.g. Ebbell, Ghalioungui and Stephan; see p. 70). These contradictory opinions continue to be disputed at the present time.

Textual evidence that shows direct translation of the earlier texts would certainly be convincing evidence, but with reference to the notion that parallel medical practices might have arisen separately in different places, it is difficult to conclude the influence of one on the other. For instance, we can find a similar manner of treatment for a dislocated jaw in Arabic books of Ibn Sina and Al Magousy and Sushruta in India (Keswani 1967: 88, 93; Ghalioungui 1969b: 165; 1973: 42), the use of liver for blindness is found in Mesopotamian medicine, the use of the root of the pomegranate is a universally found treatment against parasitic worms. Nonetheless, with regard to this difficult matter Ghalioungui (1968: 97–8) states:

> … I do not insist on the evidence of ordinary household remedies common to both countries, e.g., the common use as a cough remedy of honey, butter and cumin (Dioscorides II, 33 and Berlin Papyrus 31), or the use of honey for cough that is mentioned twelve times in the Ebers and Berlin Papyri with or without cream (Dioscorides II, 82), or the utilization against chronic cough of inhalation (Dioscorides II, 35) that the Egyptians were the first to use (Eb.325). Such coincidences may be natural in neighbouring and ecologically similar countries. But when the remedy is too unusual, or when it bears the same name, the resemblance goes far beyond the possibilities of mere chance. Among the unusual remedies we have already met with bile recommended as a treatment of eye condition by the Ebers Papyrus and the Bible, but also by Dioscorides (II, 96), Pliny, and Avicenna (V, 12). Flies' dirt was prescribed for baldness in the Ebers papyrus (Eb.782) and flies' heads in Dioscoride (I, 89) … Many other medications merit mentioning on the same account, for example calcinated hedgehogs' spines as a cure for baldness (reproduced by Dioscorides); urine as an ointment to prevent regrowth of an eyelash, or in a mixture to cure haematuria and epilepsy (the first repeated by Dioscorides, the second in addition by Pliny and the Copts). We have also crocodile dung (Eb.738) mentioned by Pliny (XXVIII, 108) as "crocodilea", beef liver for night blindness (Eb.51, London 35 and Dioscorides II, 45), and arsenic sulphide by Egyptians, Greeks and Copts. The most extraordinary of these however is a recipe in a collection of magical cures which consists of a mouse fried in oil to cure dentition trouble (Z. 8, 2–3 (Berlin

[120] Blackman (1927, reprinted in 2000: 210–11) introduces some prescriptions of folk medicine of contemporary Egypt such as a treatment for diarrhoea with leaves from a sycamore and for inflamed eyes by using the dung of a black donkey. These appear similar to the ancient Egyptian remedies.

Papyrus no. 3027)), found also in Dioscorides (II, 69) and that reached the present folklore of many European countries.

Saunders (1963: 4) also states that "However, direct influences are more clearly perceived in specific medical theories or *dogmata*, in diagnostic tests, and in therapeutic methods which involve complex manipulation or complicated formulae having some special and precise application." Here they both emphasis the significance of a peculiar practice and concept of medicine as criteria in assuming a relationship between two different medicines. It is upon this peculiarity of medicine that Stephan bases his argument for the Egyptian origin of the test for a woman's ability to conceive by use of the onion pessary and its transmission from there into other cultures: "Da dieser Test natürlich keine zutreffenden Ergebnisse liefern kann, da er auf falschen anatomischen Voraussetzungen beruht, muß hier eine Tradierung vorliegen. Diagnostische und therapeutische Maßnahmen, die auf realen Grundlagen basieren, können durch parallele Empirie gleichzeitig oder nacheinander, aber unabhängig voneinander entdeckt worden sein. Maßnahmen, die keine reproduzierbaren Ergebnisse liefern, müssen wohl tradiert worden sein." (Stephan 2005: 94) (see p. 41, 44).

The Greek and Roman medical texts often provide statements clarifying the conceptual aspects of their medical practice, which is lacking in Egyptian texts, and these are very helpful in enabling us to understand the medical theories of the Greeks. Because we are aware of the Egyptian influence on Greek medicine, scholars often assume that it may be possible to uncover significant relationships between the medical ideas of Egypt, Greece and Rome, and to this end significant comparative studies of medical texts have been undertaken.[121]

Ghalioungui (1973: 106–9) noticed several parallels in concepts of gynaecology. The Ebers papyrus (Eb.808) speaks of "The beginning of remedies not to allow that both breasts fall down. They are smeared with the blood of one whose menstruation has just begun; her belly and her thighs are rubbed therewith; *gs.w* cannot happen to her." The term *gs.w* is difficult to understand. Ebbell (1937: 110) translates it as "abortion." Ghalioungui (1987: 205) questions the meaning of the word: "Is *gs.w* related to *gsgs* 'overrun' and does it mean something like 'overflow' with milk?" and notes the supposition of a connection between the uterus (and its blood supply) and the breasts which is explicit in several Hippocratic writings: "Milk is akin to the menses when the eighth month is gone and the nutriment passes over (to the breast)" (Hip.V, 118). "If a pregnant woman's breasts suddenly become withered, she miscarriages" (Aph.V, 37). "If milk flows from the breasts of a pregnant woman, it is an indication that the foetus will be weak" (Aph.V, 52). Then Ghalioungui (1973: 106) introduces a citation of Galen's text which, as usual, has a ready explanation:

> Since she (nature) prepared both these parts (breasts and uterus) to be of service in a single work, she has joined them by many of the vessels ... (that) go to breasts, by bringing down veins and arteries to the hypochondrium and to the whole hypogastrium, and then by attaching these to the vessels which come up from the parts below and from which veins extend to the uterus. For the parts are the only ones needing to be connected by vessels in order that whenever an embryo is being formed and is growing in the uteri, it alone may be flooded with nutriment from both parts of the common veins, and in order that when the child has been born, all the nutriment may in turn flow to the breasts.

As a result, the foetus is weak if the breasts secrete milk "because of course all the surplus left in the veins by a weak foetus unable to attract enough to nourish itself suitably, rises to the breasts." Ghalioungui (1973: 106) also notes that a similar concept appears to be surmised by Celsus (1st century BC) and by Ibn Sina.

Another case of a possible understanding of an Egyptian medical concept through the comparison with the Greek and other related medicines is the Egyptian prescription "to cause a woman's womb to go to its place" (Eb.789–95). Ghalioungui (1973: 108) sees the notion of the "womb to go to its place" as comparable to the Greek's "wandering womb" or *hysteria*, where the uterus wandering around the body causes illness. According to him, the Hippocratic writings are rich in references to the movements of the womb and to the symptoms they may cause. The example (Hip.VII, 33 and 315) provided is that "if the uterus moves towards the liver, the woman loses her voice, clenches her teeth, etc., or that when it approaches the liver or the hypochondrium it causes suffocation, rolling of the eyes ... etc." This view was adopted by the physicians of a later period, and Ghalioungui (1973: 108) notes that the treatment by the Roman physician Celsus was that "to stop it, fumigations with foetid substances had to be applied and, thereafter, counter-irritation to the epigastrium." There are several methods prepared for womb moving in the Ebers papyrus, and among them two cases of fumigation treatment: "... dry excrement of men on frankincense, and the woman is fumigated therewith" (Eb.793) and "... an ibis of wax is placed on charcoal; let the fume thereof enter into the vulva ..." (Eb.795). Green (2003: 272) notices a similar treatment in the Hippocratic corpus (*Sterile Woman*): "The following treatment was indicated;

[121] Yahuda (1947: 550) emphases the significance of a comparative study between Hebrew and Egyptian medicine noting that, "the way is opened to identifying the Hebrew names of some diseases, drugs, and remedies ... whereas the Egyptian medical papyri throw a light on Biblical medicine, it is also possible to find out the true meaning of some Egyptian medical expressions, and to identify some diseases or anatomical parts of the body by establishing the Hebrew equivalent and parallels"; In the study of identifying the *nꜣnꜣ*-plant as a mint, Long (1984) notes patterns of the Egyptian use of the *nꜣnꜣ*-plant in medical papyri and reveals its association with specific ingredients, diseases and application forms, and then he demonstrates terminological and philological comparisons with Greek and Roman texts. Bardinet (1999) applies a similar methodology in the identification of the material *ḥs n ꜥff* (lit. "fly's dirt") as a propolis.

a woman should crouch over a bowel of sweet perfumes while smelling something rancid. The theory was that the uterus would be attracted to the fragrance of the perfumes, while being repelled by the stench." Concerning ailments related to the womb, we may also refer to the older texts of the Kahun papyrus such as "Instructions for a woman suffering in her neck, abdomen and her ears, she hears not what is said to her you should say concerning her: It is due to violence(?) of the womb" (Kh.8), "… a woman suffering in her urine, as though expressing the fluid of a discharge … it is defluxions(?) of the womb" (Kh.10) or "… a woman who loves bed, she does not rise and does not shake it … it is spasms(?) of the womb" (Kh.11).[122]

The studies by Stueur *et al.* (1959) and Saunders (1963) suggest the transmission of Egyptian faecal pathology into Greek medicine. Saunders (1963: 22) states:

> The fundamental concept of residue as a primary aetiological factor in loss of health initiated by the Egyptians became common among Greek physicians and was greatly elaborated by them. We find it in its simpler and original form in the teachings of the older physicians, especially in the reported views of Euryphon, the founder of the Cnidian School, Herodicos of Cnidos, and Alcamenes of Abydos (Papyrus Anonymus Londinensis IV, 31 ff), it is perhaps not by chance that closer reflection of Egyptian theory should exist among the members of the older school at Cnidos, since the Cnidians were nearer in time to Egyptian practices.

Certainly, there are many difficulties apparent in the comparison of faecal pathology from Egypt and Greece, partly due to the paucity of explanatory texts in the Egyptian medical papyri and partly due to the diversity of views concerning faecal pathology held by the Greeks. Nonetheless, important textual evidence which may reveal the conceptual similarity between the Egyptian and Greek is found in the Papyrus Anonymus Londinensis of the Cnidian school of medicine. Steuer *et al.* (1959: 27) gives a text of this papyrus (IV, 31–40):

> Euryphon of Cnidus, for example, thinks that diseases are caused in the following manner. "When the belly does not discharge the nutriment that has been taken, residues are produced, which then rise to the regions about the head and cause diseases. When however the belly is empty and clean, digestion takes place as it should; otherwise what I have already stated occurs.

This statement explains the notion of faecal pathology where the residue results from an excess of food in the bowel and the abnormal conditions of digestion, and the teaching of Herodicu of Cnidus in this papyrus (V, 6–10) mentions that the residue which "lies undigested and unaltered in the belly" would lead to being "transformed into *περίττωμα* (*perittōma*)" (Steuer *et al.* 1959: 24). The term *perittōma* in Cnidian medicine is the crucial faecal pathogen which is generated from the faecal residue that causes various diseases through its putrefactive power; and scholars consider that the Greek notion of *perittōma* is comparable to the Egyptian *wḫdw*.[123] A diagnostic text of the Berlin papyrus (Bln.154) is provided for comparison: "… if he crouches in order to evacuate (then) his intestines are under pressure, (but) he is not getting along with the evacuation. You should say concerning him; this is one who is under a pool of *wḫdw* in his body; he feels his heart; he is sick (and) I shall act (on his behalf). Should it rise in him and become an occlusion, you will have to apply remedies against *wḫdw*, together with remedies to destroy *wḫdw*" (Steuer *et al.* 1959: 38).[124]

A similar notion of the faecal pathology is also found in the Hippocratic corpus (e.g. *On Regimen* VI, 612) and also other Greek medical texts (e.g. Aristotle *Meteorologica* 381b, 12ff) (Saunders 1963: 22–4), but making a precise comparison of the conceptual links is problematic due to the enigmatic variations and differences showed in the pathological descriptions in the texts. Nonetheless, studies could bring to light some more hypothetical conceptual correspondences in the Egyptian and Greek medical texts, although, as usual, there are many disagreements. Saunders (1963: 29–30) notes that an inflammatory skin lesion resulting from the putrefactive residue mentioned in the Greek texts (e.g. *On Diseases* IV) corresponds to the purulent skin diseases called *šfwt* and *wḥ3w* brought from *wḫdw*. For the identification of the Egyptian term *stt* and *ʿrwt*, Ebbell (1937: 25–6) looks closely for a correspondence with Greek medical writings:

> For the word *stt* is used in various places in a way showing that it must have been an analogue of the Greek *φλέγμα* (Phlegm): it is sometimes determined as a fluid, it may putrify (sic) and may make its way to different organs, producing diseases in them, and just the same ailments as are alleged to be brought about by phlegm, e.g. ileus (see Papyrus Ebers 25, 3–8 and the Hippocratic work "de glandulis" chap. 14). Further, some terms in the Papyrus Ebers have led me to suppose that the word *ʿrwt* may possibly correspond to the Greek *χολή* (Bile).

In the last part of the introduction to his translation of the Ebers papyrus, Ebbell (1937: 25–6) insists conclusively

[122] Ghalioungui (1967a: 41) also observes concerning the expression "the wind of the pest of the year" that refers to an epidemic in the Edwin Smith papyrus (Sm.verso.XVIII, 1) that "Cette acception s'apparente à la notion grecque des 'miasmata' que Galien pensait être des particules dans l'air qui pouvaient provoquer des fièvres pestilentielles"; See p. 26.

[123] Prioreschi (2003: 152) notes the persistence of the notion of faecal pathology until relatively recently: "The concept of a toxic material absorbed from the intestine as a cause of disease was to persist in Western medical thought until modern time in the notions about the etiology of puerperal fever of the prebacteriological era and in the theory of 'autointoxication' of the 19th and early 20th century."

[124] Long (1984: 148) employs the term "*περίττωμα*" as a translation for *wḫdw*.

that "it must then at once be pointed out that Greek medicine is by no means so original as people were formerly inclined to believe, but that a very great deal of it has been taken over from the ancient Egyptians ... and can only be looked upon as a further development of the latter."[125] In accordance with this conviction he translated many Egyptian words based on Greek medical notions and terms. The term *stt*, for instance, starts with the Hieroglyph representing an animal skin pierced by an arrow 𓄜 (Gardiner sign-list: F 29) and ends with the pus determinative, and it appears to be related to the verb *st* which means "shoot" or "pierce," probably expressing "shooting pains" as Dawson (1934: 185–8) suggests.[126] The characteristic symptomatic descriptions of disease related to *stt* seems to be acute pain and stiffness of the limbs (Eb.295–6). Ebbell (1937: 64) then interprets *stt* as rheumatism, reasoning that "The Egyptian word '*śtt*' is used both as a designation for rheumatism or rheumatic pains and as the name of the 'phlegm,' one of the disease-producing humours. Probably the Egyptians thought that rheumatism was due to this humour, and thus designated both of them by the same word. The primary sense of '*śtt*' is possibly the same as that of the Greek 'rheuma', viz. a flow, a flux." [127] Ebbell's interpretations and translations, however, are often considered to be over-enthusiastic and speculative and meet heavy criticism from other scholars.[128]

The comparative study of medicine is highly problematic. Noticing a similarity alone does not allow us to confirm an actual correlation of the medicines of different cultures. One can only speculate as to whether "On the Heart" written by Diocles (350 BC) describing cardiac value might have been a text which originally came from Egypt (Cave 1950: 570), or one may think that the Egyptian *gs-tp* (Eb.250; lit. "half-head"; i.e. modern *migraine*) was later rendered as ἡμικρανία in Greece (Latin *hemikrania*) (Harris 1971: 117; Westendorf 1999: 141; Pahor 2003: 1357–8).[129] Steuer *et al.* (1959: 55) describes the difficulties encountered by comparative study of medicine:

> At the same time, it should be recognized that interpretation is exceedingly difficult in such subtle matters as the endeavor to seek causal explanations of disease. Interpretation is especially difficult, too, because the terms are so extremely labile, with great overlap in meaning: *wḫdw*, *ḥs* and *ṯsw*; perittōma, kopros, phlegm and bile. Likewise, it should not be forgotten that with the translation to newer theories older terms were retained that, though they had new meanings, tended to carry over to a varying extent the fundamental ideas associated with the old.

4.3 Egyptian medicine as pre-rational medicine

Some scholars such as Ebbell, emphasise the significant indications for Egyptian influence on Greek medicine and regard Greek medicine as a continuation of Egyptian medicine. But other scholars such as Staden consider that the Egyptian influence was necessarily limited to the primitive practices of medicine, if any. Concerning assertions of the Egyptian influence on Greek medicine, Staden (1989: 3) comments:

> The enduring nature of this Greek esteem, combined with the relatively high standards displayed in parts of Egyptian medical papyri of Pharaonic times, has prompted modern claims that the debt of Greek medicine to Pharaonic Egypt was considerable. Moreover, it has been suggested that the efflorescence of scientific medicine in Alexandria in the third century B.C. is attributable in large measure to the Alexandrian physicians' direct exposure to native Egyptian medicine. These views have, however, also met with radical scepticism.

Three factors that he (1989: 4–5) points out are (1) the chronological gap between the time of Egyptian medical papyri and the Greek period, (2) the lexicographical and philological difficulties which impede a conclusive answer to the question and (3) the occurrence of a similar general notion in different cultures. These are difficulties which have been noted above.[130] His methods of comparison

---

125 See also Ebbell (1928: 115), Westendorf (1999: 344, n.527) and Stephan (2005: 97).

126 Westendorf's (1999: 343) translation of *stt* as "Schleimstoffe" is based on the term *sti* which means "strömen, gießen" and the water determinative attached in two cases; See p. 33.

127 Saunders (1963: 24): "As to whether the Egyptian terms *ʿrwt* and *stt* refer respectively to bile and phlegm, as suggested by Ebbell, is still conjectural, but it is clear that, whatever these terms specifically mean, the objects they refer to also undergo corruption, bringing about pathological conditions"; Stephan (2005: 93) states on *stt*, which he translates as "Schleimstoffe", that "Sie haben in der griechischen Medizin offenbar ein Pendant im Phlegma, einem Schleimstoff, der zwar nicht im Magen entsteht, aber die gleichen Eigenschaften besitzt wie die ägyptischen Schleimstoffe, und zusammen mit der Galle in der hippokratischen Schrift *De morbo sacro* eine Zweisäftelehre bildet, die dann unter dem Einfluß der Vierelementenlehre des Empedokles im Corpus Hippokraticum zur Viersäftelehre (Blut, Schleim, dunkle Galle, helle Galle) ausgebaut wird."

128 One reason that Ebbell's interpretation is mentioned as being speculative is that he tries to associate many different elements to formulate an identification. Temkin (1938: 126–31), for instance, criticises Ebbell's interpretation of *nsjt* as "epilepsy." He mentions this identification is arrived at because in the Ebers papyrus (Eb.201) the *nsjt* is compared to *hjt* which he thinks connote cramps, and the Berlin papyrus (Eb.112) attributes *nsjt* to the influence of demons, and this, to Ebbell, points to epilepsy; and he sees final confirmation in the fact that the remedies against *nsjt* are partly magic, such as incantations and also the use of substances prescribed against epilepsy by Greek and Roman authors.

129 Pahor (2003: 1357) also notes that a reference to a "malady of half the head" has the same meaning in Arabic—*sodah nesf al-raas*.

130 The chronological gap certainly creates a difficulty when associating medicines of different epochs. But the fact of historical transmission of medicine, as seen in Greek medicine to Arabs and Europe and in the continuity of Chinese and Indian medicine, indicates that a medicine could be transmitted over centuries (see Chapter 2). Jouanna (2004: 2) states "on se posa la question de la relation qu'il pouvait y avoir entre cette médecine égyptinne … et la première production médicale grecque ... L'écart considerable de la chronologie n'est pas en soi un obstacle majeur à la comparaison, puisque la médecine égyptienne dans les papyrus conserves s'étale sur une longue période

of Egyptian and Greek medicine, however, are quite different as he describes Egyptian medicine necessarily as primitive. One reason he thinks Egyptian medicine is primitive is the occasional accompanying incantations with the prescriptions. Staden (1989: 4–6) states:

> The amalgam of magic, law, and empiricism that characterizes the medicine of the Pharaohs ... as late as the second century A.D., Egyptian pharmacology is still associated with magic spells and incantations, which indeed are richly represented in Pharaonic medical papyri. When medical theories and practices are supported and sanctioned by ritual, by belief in magic, and by the priesthood, they can become relatively immune to the revisionary processes that tend to be associated with scientific growth ...

He then introduces the few Egyptian incantations from medical papyri that infer religious and mythological notions, together with the other practices of Egyptian magical therapy.[131] According to Staden (1989: 6) the "pervasive magico-religious dimension of Egyptian medicine is largely foreign both to Alexandrian and to pre-Alexandrian Greek medicine." He does not deny, however, that there is ample evidence for magico-religious forms of therapy in the Greek culture, especially from the Hellenistic period, and he also observes that there is no evidence for the Greek physicians ever objecting to the priestly assistance offered at the temple of Asclepius (Staden 1989: 8). Nonetheless, he notes that "Alexandrian and Hippocratic medicine appear to eschew the spells, incantations, and charms which dominate many—and intrude upon all—Pharaonic medical papyri," and the significant difference between the two cultures that he points out is that "In Greek society, priest and physician exercised their distinct functions in sharply different ways, even if they shared the same god; in Egypt many medical practitioners were also priests of the goddess Sekhmet ..." (1989: 8–9). In the last paragraph of his introduction, he concludes "In medicine, being 'Hellenistic' or 'Alexandrian', as opposed to 'archaistic' or 'Egyptian', clearly entailed being considerably more advanced in theory, and probably in practice as well" (Staden 1989: 31).

allant des années 1800 jusqu'à une époque postérieure à Hippocrate, l'époque ptolémaïque, sans que l'on perçoive une evolution majeure"; A discussion concerning conservative transmission of medicine in ancient Egypt is presented in Chapter 5.

[131] Fraser (1972: 344–5) also considers that the influence of Egyptian medicine on Greek medicine was only limited to the primitive practice of Egyptian medicine, stating that: "... there can be no doubt that Greek medicine adopted traditional Egyptian lore at an early date. Nevertheless, this age-old practice, even at its best, does not seem to have advanced beyond observation and treatment, and Egyptian civilization showed in this, as in many other respects, its chronic inability to draw inferences and establish general principles from practical knowledge ... Thus it seems that the debt of the professional Alexandrian anatomists of the third century, with their lively Greek tradition of medical science, to the native Egyptian tradition may be discounted as negligible."

Integrity of science and religion in ancient Egypt

Staden's arguments are convincing in some respects, but his statements necessitate us to reconsider the "medico-magical" aspect of Egyptian medical practice and also the ways in which modern thinking differs from antiquity in recognising what is "scientific" and "religious." Staden regards healing by means of incantations as essentially a "religious" practice of an archaic culture that is contrary to the "scientific" rational medicine of an advanced culture. But I know of no culture without religion, and healing is always based on some form of religious notion whether in ancient or modern societies or in western or eastern cultures, although there may be some differences in the degree of reliance and preference or in the occupation of the persons who practice healing. Also, just as considerable evidence reveals the extensive use of magic by the Greeks, or even by Galen who commonly practiced healing with amulets, so we can still find similar practices in modern civilized societies.

Some Egyptian incantations referred to by Staden (1989: 6–7) come from the Ebers papyrus, and indeed, they exhibit the characteristic features of Egyptian religion and myth, including the names of divinities such as the gods Ra, Osiris, Isis and Horus, and the recitations are mostly reflections of mythological stories. Such incantations may give the impression of an archaic religion and strange ethnic practices. But Dawson (1964: 70–2) notes that in other cultures also the practice of interspersing incantations among prescriptions is very similar to that found in the Egyptian documents, although the names of Horus, Isis and the lesser divinities invoked in the papyri are replaced by those of Christ, the Virgin Mary and the Christian Saints, in addition, at the end of the prescriptions the words are often added "tried and found perfect," "probatum," etc. just as in the Egyptian texts. Nonetheless, the point to make here is that incantations (or other forms of magical healing) are a form of medicine that was incorporated into the medical pluralism of a culture, and its practice, originating in the remote past and by no means extinct in the present, should not be confused with other aspects of medicine.[132] With the ancient Egyptians, we can establish a clear distinction between treatments by remedies and those made by incantation, as stated in an incantation of the Ebers papyrus (Eb.3): "Strong is *ḥkꜣ* (lit. "magic"; i.e. incantation) over *pẖrt* ("remedy") and vice-versa."[133]

[132] Karenberg *et al.* (2001: 915) states "... most patients throughout the centuries, regardless of the actual mainstream opinion in medicine, relied on healers who had an intimate connection with supernatural forces" and notes that the best example from Christian civilization is Saint Denis or Saint Denni who plays an important role as a patron saint for all sufferers from headache.

[133] Leitz (2005: 43) notes "Es soll im folgenden plausible gemacht werden, daß die Opposition des Satzes vom Anfang des Papyrus Ebers, also die zwischen *ḥkꜣ* und *pẖrt* nicht auf der Ebene Magie versus Nichtmagie zu suchen ist: Gemeint ist vielmehr die zwischen dem gesprochenen, vielleicht nur gemurmelten Zauberspruch und dem tatsächlichen, auf jeden Fall materiellen Heilmittel, das hergestellt, eingenommen,

However, a close relationship may have existed between the incantation and remedy as far as the principles and theory of medicine are concerned that they are based on, particularly when the ailments to be treated were considered to have resulted from demonical aetiology. Staden asserts that the "scientific" mind of the Greek physicians is demonstrated by (what he regards as) their avoidance of incantations. He also provides scientific aspects of Greek medical writings:

> Thus the Hippocratic treatise *On Sacred Disease*, with its criticism of magic and with its overt questioning of etiologies that resort to the divine, is known to practically all historians of ancient science ... Privileging, historiographically, Hippocratic methodological debates (*On Ancient Medicine*), criticisms of magic (*On Sacred Disease*), impressively detailed observational accounts (*Epidemics*), and attempts at measurement and quantification over the 'irrational' or 'folkloristic' or 'magical' within Hippocratic writings ... —all such acts of privileging might make eminent sense from the point of view of a modern version of 'science' (Staden 1992: 584).

In *On Sacred Disease*, the notion of the "Sacred disease" which considered epilepsy to be caused by a god, is negated, and the magical treatments against this disease are criticised as being due to ignorance of how to treat it.[134] And in the text the author argues "this disease seems to me to be no more divine than any other disease. It has the same nature as others, and the same cause," providing his own view: "now this disease attacks the phlegmatic, but not the bilious ... there is no need to put it in a special category and to consider it more divine than other disease; they are all divine, and all human" (*On Sacred Disease*, 8–21; Chadwick 1978: 242–50). Such statements of negation of demonical aetiology and criticism of the "magical" treatments practiced by colleagues appeals to our modern sense of the "scientific," in contrast to the "religious."[135] This clear recognition of a "scientific" aspect contrasting with a "religious" aspect, however, cannot be properly applied to Egyptian religion and science due to their integrity.[136]

Before we consider the scientific aspects of ancient Egyptian religion, it is necessary to discuss the difficult concept of "magic." A primitive type of magic can be aptly understood as any action that is aimed at and intends to achieve an immediate goal through the simple and limited conceptual assumption of cause and effect.[137] But a significant advance is made towards the concept of "magic" when its principle is based on the concept of the regularity of the universe. It would then no longer be an attitude of arbitrary recognition of phenomenal facts as in primitive magic but become an attentive participation in and operation of the laws of the universe. A clearer indication of the Egyptian's recognition of the significance of the regularity of universe can be found in the creation myth whose description expresses the idea that the universe began from an unordered, inert watery Abyss (*nun*) through the establishment of the order of the universe (*mꜣꜥt*).[138] In the myth, more specifically, the sun god Ra appears as the

aufgelegt oder sonst irgendwie appliziert wird"; Walker (1990: 85) states "their existence does not signify that there was a 'rational,' empirical stream of Egyptian medical practice parallel to a non-rational magical stream. Magical incantations in the papyri sometimes stand on their own but many occur in association with a prescription-remedy or a case-study; not alongside them as mere accompaniments but integrated into them to form a composite whole. In any particular clinical situation, Egyptian physicians were not compelled to choose one system of treatment over the other. Pharmacological prescriptions and magical incantations belonged to a single coherent and consistent system of medical theory and practice and both were delivered by the same practitioner."

[134] The author of *On the Sacred Disease* states, "in making use, too, of purifications and incantations they do what I think is a very unholy and irreligious thing. For the suffers from the disease they purify with blood and such like, as though they are polluted ... All such they ought to have treated in the opposite way ... yet if a god is indeed the cause, they ought to have taken them to the sanctuaries and offered them to him."

[135] King (2001: 7) notes that when the author of *On the Sacred Disease* criticises the name of "the sacred disease," he does not deny that it is "divine," but he insists instead that it is no more "divine" than other diseases; We may also note that he is criticising the use of incantation not as "irrational" but as "unholy" and "irreligious," indicating that he is not denying the religion itself.

[136] Leitz (2005: 42–3) makes the following observations about co-existence of the medicinal and magical treatments in Egyptian papyri: "In Wirklichkeit handelt es sich jedoch bei der Vorstellung, man könne für das alte Ägypten eine Trennung zwischen medizinischen und magischen Texten durchführen, um eine Fiktion. Es ist methodisch nicht sehr glücklich, eine moderne Einteilung der Wissenschaftsgebiete in die Vergangenheit zu transponieren und dann getrennte Korpora beispielsweise von medizischen, magischen, astronomischen und anderen Texten aufzustellen, die in der Antike selbst jedoch eine Einheit bilden konnten. Hinzu kommt, daß es auch auf der sozialen Ebene in vielen Fällen keine Trennung zwischen Arzt und Zauberer gab, oft handelte es sich um die gleichen Personen, die nur unterschiedliche Titel trugen."

[137] Ritner (2001a: 321) states "The concept of 'magic' has proved to be a most difficult category for modern Egyptology, with little agreement regarding the definition or scope of supposedly magical practices. The designation of 'magic' has been applied subjectively to any actions or recitations deemed 'non-religious' by individual authors. Following the early anthropological theories of James G. Frazer (*The Golden Bough*, 1910) and Bronislaw Malinowski (*Magic, Science and Religion and Other Essays*, 1948), 'magic' is most frequently distinguished from 'religion' on the basis of the former's 'blasphemous,' threatening attitude (as opposed to 'proper' humanity) and its immediate, limited, and personal goals (contrasted with rites and prayers for general well-being). Unfortunately, such distinctions are inadequate for ancient Egypt, where a threatening attitude may be adopted in orthodox public rituals for general benefit, and identical texts and rites may serve either personal or general ends. Seeking to avoid this problem 'magico-religious,' while others have urged the abandonment of any category of magic. A working definition of *magic* as 'any activity which seeks to obtain its goal by methods outside the simple cause and effect' has been proposed by Ritner (1993, p.69) and adopted in subsequent reference works (M. Depouw, *A Companion to Demotic Studies*, Brussels, 1997, p.109)."

[138] Teeter (2001: 319) states "The ethical conceptions of 'truth', 'order', and 'cosmic balance' are encompassed in the Egyptian term *maat*, and the personification of those principles is the goddess Maat (*mꜣꜥt*). The goddess represented the divine harmony and balance of the universe, including the unending cycles of the rising and setting of the sun, the inundation of the Nile River, the resulting fertility of the land, and the enduring office of kingship; she was considered to be the force that kept chaos (*isft*), the antithesis of order, from overwhelming the world. Hence *maat* was a complex, intertwined, and interdependent sense of ethics that tied personal behaviour—such as speaking truthfully, dealing fairly in the market place, and especially sustaining obedience to parents, the king, and his agents—to the maintenance of universal order."

primeval creator of the universe,[139] and he engenders the god Shu (divinity of air) and the goddess Tefnut (divinity of moisture), and these divinities in turn bring forth the god Geb (divinity of earth) and the goddess Nut (divinity of sky),[140] and these cosmogenic divinities play roles in maintaining the stability and harmony of the universe, *mꜣꜥt*.[141] The Egyptian religious texts often illustrate and emphasise the regularity of celestial movements, the annual flooding of the Nile or any other natural phenomena, and are understood through the attribution of divine forces.[142] It is *ḥkꜣ* (i.e. magic) that the divinities use to maintain nature in order and balance. Such myths may appear to us merely as ethnic illustrations of ancient mythological notions, but they are not entirely irrelevant to the actual study of astronomy and the observations of other natural phenomena.[143] We may think the Egyptian mythological expression of annual cycles together with the Egyptians' establishment of the calendar of 365 days as reflecting their attentive and scientific attitudes to the observation of nature.[144] Another significant observation concerning the perception of universal order is the fact that abnormal and disastrous phenomena, which in primitive magic were arbitrarily recognised as individual situations particular to them to be dealt, are understood as resulting from disturbances in order and harmony brought about by some causes.[145] Thus magic is a tool to eliminate disturbance and restore the order and harmony of the cosmos.[146] It was also the primary duty of the king to maintain the order of the universe through upholding *mꜣꜥt* and through services to the divinities, and at the same time, it was the kings' upholding of *mꜣꜥt* that established Egyptian kingship, which, in turn, maintained the order of society.[147] There was a principle of macrocosm and microcosm where the law of the universe can be related to the stability and security of the society. The king was at the centre and the force of *mꜣꜥt*, and the people were obligated to follow this *mꜣꜥt*, and thus the term *mꜣꜥt* is often aptly translated as "justice" or "truth" in a social context.[148] In ancient Egypt, therefore, *mꜣꜥt* is the truth of the universe, and it is a genuine science, achieved through attentive observations of every part of natural phenomena, to realize and understand the mysterious order of universe. It is the socio-political science to understand the divine order of the universe and its relationship, via the *mꜣꜥt* of kingship, to the structure and functioning of the society. Egyptian performance of magic is based on the holy knowledge of *mꜣꜥt* and is scientific to them. Thus eliminating the concept of divinity and divine influence or the negation of religion

139 In Egyptian creation mythology, emphasis is placed on Ra's coming into being at the beginning of time. For the acts of creation, Ra coalesces with this aspect of the sun-god, e.g., Khnum, Amun, Atum and Khepri (Hart 1986: 179–80).

140 The Heliopolitan Ennead (Nine Gods) consists of the sun-god creator and his descendants: Shu, Tefnut, Geb, Nut, Osiris, Isis, Seth and Nephthys (Hart 1986: 65).

141 A complex conceptionalization of *mꜣꜥt* is exhibited in the Egyptian religious texts. In Egyptian religion, *mꜣꜥt* can appear to be a personified deity regarded as a daughter of the creator sun god. Assmann (1990: 163) notes her role as being a force to direct correct process: "... dann ist Ma`at als Tochter des Sonnengottes die Kraft, die dem Sonnenlauf seine Richtung gibt. Damit aber hält sie die Welt insgesamt in Gang; denn der Sonnenlauf ist nach ägyptischer Vorstellung der Kosmos, der vom Ägypter nicht als Raum, sondern als Prozeß gedacht wird ... Ma`at wirkt lenkend, hier wie dort, indem sie den Prozeß in den richtigen Bahnen hält und zum Gelingen steuert. Ma`at ist eine regulative Energie, die das Leben der Menschen zur Eintracht, Gemeinsamkeit und Gerechtigkeit steuert und die kosmischen Kräfte zur Gesetzmäßigkeit ihrer Bahnen, Rhythmen und Wirkungen ausbalanciert"; Different aspects represented by the *mꜣꜥt* is also reflected in the incantations for healing which recite "... I am *mꜣꜥt*, the daughter of Re ..." (BM EA 10309) and "Hail to you, that son of Ra, whom Atum himself engendered ... he of *mꜣꜥt*, load of *mꜣꜥt* ..." (BM EA 10042) (Leitz 1999: 29, 32).

142 For example, adoration of Ra in his rising, crossing of the sky and resting in the horizon of the western mountains each day is expressed in the hymn to the rising sun, and blessings of annual flood are exhibited in a hymn to the god of the inundating Nile, Hapy, who "anchors the earthly rhythms, returning in his due season" (Lichtheim 1973: 204–10; Foster 2001: 110–19).

143 Dunand *et al.* states "Since the gods were phenomenological realities that belonged to the physics of the universe, and in this regard were immanent in it, it was absurd to believe or not believe in their existence" (2004: 6) and emphases that the Egyptians explained "physical phenomena mythologically, with superhuman powers called gods" (2004: 159).

144 The establishment of the calendar of 365 days requires attentive and continuous observations of the celestial movement, and this cannot be achieved in one generation but requires systematic observation over the course of generations. Thus there must have been written records of observed celestial movements, based on which calculations were operated by later generations, although none of them have come down to us. This would illustrate the scientific mind and the practice of science of the ancient Egyptians; On the adjustments of the calendar that occurred in ancient Egypt, see Parker (1952).

145 An example of a treatment based on primitive arbitrary magical ideas is mentioned in Chapter 2 (see p. 10).

146 Walker (1990: 90) states "They had experienced and overcome every adversity that could ever befall a human being: natural disaster, accident, illness, legal accusation, murderous assault, and so on. They had triumphed over these adversities by means of their magic power (*ḥkꜣ*). Amongst the gods, Isis and Thoth were the most knowledgeable about magic and were the most skilled practitioners of its art. After all the struggles had been waged, the defeats suffered and the victories won in this mythical First Time, the mechanisms for resolving disorders of every description had been learned and the pattern for the orderly working of the universe (that is, for *mꜣꜥt*) had been established. Any calamity in the real world, such as a serious illness, was believed to threaten the continued harmonious working of the entire cosmos. To restore order and harmony the magician/physician had to magically conjure the analogous calamity and outcome that had occurred during the mythical First Time."

147 Teeter (2001: 319) states "One of the primary duties of the king was to maintain the order of the cosmos, effected by upholding the principle of *maat* through correct and just rule and through service to the gods, in turn, the people of Egypt had an obligation to uphold *maat*, through obedience to the king, who served as the intermediary between the divine and profane spheres. The *Instructions of Kagemni* record 'do *maat* for the king, for *maat* is what the king loves'; the negative confession that was recited by the deceased, as his or her soul was judged against *maat*, included the profession 'I have not disputed the king.' The sense of fealty to the king and its association with personal responsibility for the balance of the universe may help explain why there are so few periods of social unrest in Egypt—for to act against the king was to risk the stability of the cosmos. The association of government and *maat* reached even the lower levels of government. Viziers who dispensed justice in the name of the king wore a pendant in the form of the goddess Maat, which both alluded to their association with the goddess and their inspiration to act justly."

148 Concerning the homology of cosmic and social order in the spectrum of *mꜣꜥt*, Assmann (1999: 33–4) points out that "Die Frage ist nur, ob hier der Kern und der Ursprung des Ma`at –Begriffes getroffen sind," and he assumes the situation where the concept of social order is projected onto the universe, i.e. that "daß die Idee der Ma`at vielmehr im Sozialen und Ethischen verankert ist und als Kernbedeutung nicht 'Weltordnung', sondern vielmer 'Gerechtigkeit' anzusetzen ist." Assmann (1999: 167) notes "Die Vorstellung der Schöpfungsordnung gehört also in den Zusammenhang nicht des Kosmologischen, sondern des politischen Denken der Ägypter ... Das politische Handeln des Königs wird als Wiederholung und Fortsetzung der Schöpfung interpretiert."

and magical property would not make anything appear to be "scientific" to the ancient Egypt.[149]

Another minor point to mention is that the empiricism or magico-religious features recognised in Egyptian medicine are necessarily hypothetical. One can find that the prescriptions of many cultures are similar. They can include both effective herbs and impure substances, just as in the Egyptian prescriptions.[150] Even the pharmacopeia of the Royal College of Physicians of London for 1651 AD recommends such materials as hare's brain, swallow's nest, horn of the stag, rhinoceros, powdered Egyptian mummy, blood of the cat, pig, bull and tortoise, excrement of doves, goats, stallions, cows and men, bile of pigs, hawk, bulls and dears, urine of goats, boars and boys, stone from the human bladder, and dead man's fat and skull (Comrie 1909: 124; Krause 1933: 272). If such prescriptions are to be interpreted, without knowing the pharmacological theory behind them, through the "empirico-rational" and "magico-religious" perspectives they will naturally appear to be empiric and religious and be understood as primitive. We should remember that the Egyptian theories of medicine remain shrouded in veils of silence.

All that said, Staden is right to say that we should regard Greek medicine as "Hellenistic." In a differentiated view, Ebbell regards Greek medicine as a direct continuation of Egyptian medicine. However, although Greek medicine may have been strongly influenced by Egyptian medicine and may have been largely based on it, Greek medicine is essentially "Hellenistic" and should be clearly distinguished from "Egyptian." Thus, we should recognise Pharaonic, Coptic, Greek and Alexandrian medicine as essentially separate medicines though there may be strong associations among them.[151] In art, for instance, we can find the influence of the virtuosity of Egypt on archaic Greek sculpture and architecture, but we can subsequently also witness the magnificent transformation of artistic style from the idealized formalism of Egyptian art to the realism of Greek art. Similarly, in Greek narrative myths, we can find Hellenistic features derived from the original Egyptian religious notions. Thus the frequent modifications through transmission and inclusion of new elements as a result of cultural interaction make the essential distinction of the two closely related cultures necessary. A new element, which characterises Greek medicine, appears together with the faecal pathology in a statement in the Papyrus Anonymus Londinensis (IV, 26–8) that "... some have said that diseases arise because of the residues from nutriment, others hold that they are due to the elements ...," i.e. the Four-Humour theory based on concept of four elements (Saunders 1963: 22).[152] Ghalioungui (1973: 58) provides us with a fair description of the relationship between the Egyptian faecal pathology and the Four-Humour theory of Greek medicine:

> The concept of disease spreading through the vessels and being eliminated in the excreta seems to herald the theory of humours. Nevertheless, one can find nowhere in Pharaonic Egypt the Classic Hippocratic notion of humoral constitution, based on the theory that the four humours are normal constituents of the body, that their harmonious blending is the basis of health, and that disharmony constitutes disease. This is far removed from the *st.t*, *r.wt*, and *wḫdw*, that are purely morbid factors. But since the early works of the Corpus Hippocraticum still understood phlegm and bile in the Cnidian sense, i.e. as pathogenic fluxions, the humoral theory may have started on these bases, although it could have developed only after a long maturation in the mathematical and cosmological context of Greek thought.[153]

149 Modern science is characterized by its discipline of reproducible evidence in the planned observations to test hypotheses and the significance of regularity in the tested result.

150 Prioreschi (2003: 157) mentions that a patient consulting a Greek physician had probably no greater chances of being helped than one consulting an Egyptian physician: "The Hippocratic treatment of baldness (cataplasm of cumin, pigeon's dung, horse-radish, leek, beet, nettle) (*On Women's Diseases* II, 189) was surely not more effective than the one advocated in the Ebers papyrus (mixture of fat of lion, hippopotamus, crocodile, cat, serpent, and ibex) (Eb.465). On the other hand, a very effective procedure still used today, that is, the manoeuvre for the reduction of a dislocated mandible, is found both in the Hippocratic Corpus (*On Joints* 30) and in the Smith Papyrus (Sm.25)"; Prioreschi (1993) makes a comparison of the treatments for similar cases of skull trauma found in the Edwin Smith papyrus and the Hippocratic corpus (*On Wounds in the Head*) in terms of effectiveness and safety, and concludes that assertions of the superiority of the Greek surgeons would not be appropriate.

151 Gammal (1989: 724) notes that when the Ptolemies came to the throne in Alexandria in 323 BC, they built a huge academy on the same system as in the Greek homeland and were teaching in the Greek language instead of Egyptian. At the same time, the Egyptian academies annexed to the ancient temples remained, performing their sacred duties in the preservation of the ancient Egyptian heritage in the cities of Heliopolis, Memphis, Sais, Abydos, Thebes and many others, with Egyptians, written in the Demotic script, being the main teaching language. This fact can also show the clear distinction of the two medical traditions.

152 Steuer (1948: 31) observes that "It is a task that still remains to be accomplished to elaborate further—apart from the *wḫdw* concept—on *stt*, a term of Egyptian humoral pathology previously mentioned. A critical analysis of the term will show that it is more related with *wḫdw* and its putrefaction than with phlegm (*φλέγμα*) in the sense of the Hippocratic humoral theory. As there are no other terms known Egyptian medical texts which could be successfully compared with important characteristics of the Hippocratic humoral theory—like yellow and black bile, crasis, discrasia, pepsis—there is no evidence thus far for its origin from ancient Egyptian sources."

153 In an earlier article, Ghalioungui (1960: 301) states the same opinion but specifically notes the development made through "un long mûrissement à la faveur des idées mathématiques et cosmogoniques de Pythagore, d'Alcméon (Littré, 34) et, finalement, d'Hippocrate"; A discussion of the contribution of the Pythagorean notion of mathematics and cosmology to the formation of Hippocratic medicine is made in Chapter 6.

PART 2

Investigation

This section is devoted to the issue of two premises that needed to be considered in assessing the viability of employing a statistical approach to Egyptian medical papyri. We first consider whether the Egyptian medical papyri can be regarded as representative of ancient Egyptian medicine in order for them to qualify as appropriate sample bodies for statistical operations. In the following section we will consider the poly-pharmacological principles that are needed to understand the poly-pharmacological aspect of Egyptian prescriptions and for the interpretation of the statistical patterns derived from them.

CHAPTER 5

Papyrus Ebers as a Sample Body

5.1 Medical papyri as conglomerations

We now return to discuss the main intentions of this work. The first premise we need to consider before applying statistical analysis to the Egyptian medical papyri concerns the validity of the Egyptian medical papyri as sample bodies for such an analysis. Ideally, in statistics, we expect a sample body to be consistent in its content and to be representative of the entire population. It is difficult to determine whether or not the Egyptian medical papyri are representative of the entire body of Egyptian medicine, but when we consider the fact that the Papyrus Anonymus Londinensis mentions twenty medical authorities, all of whom subscribe to the idea, and that the Hippocratic corpus consists of sixty or so different sources, varying widely in date and with topics ranging from diseases and surgery to regimens of good diets, showing diverse ideas and occasional contradictory opinions and also that the *Samhitās* of *Caraka* and *Suśruta* of India contain numerous references to an earlier period characterised by a great diversity of opinions,[154] we may feel justified in concluding that the Egyptian medical writings were composed from different sources and contain diverse medical ideas. In fact, many of the medical writings of many cultures are large amalgamated bodies of medicine of different origins, and a careful study of the Egyptian medical texts reveals that this also applies to the Egyptian medical papyri.

Most of the Egyptian medical papyri are dated to the New Kingdom, but a text found in the Ebers papyrus (Eb.856a) and the Berlin papyrus (Bln.163a) states that the writing has been found under the feet of (a statue of) the god Anubis at the time of King Usaphais (Den). Another text in the Ebers papyrus (Eb.468) mentions a remedy that is made for the lady Shesh, the mother of King Athothis (Djer). Since both Usaphais and Athothis are the kings of the 1st Dynasty, 5th and 3rd king respectively, we can assume that these texts were composed in the early Dynastic Period. The London papyrus (Lo.25b) includes a paragraph that describes a remarkable story, according to which the text was "found at night, having fallen into the hand of a lector priest in the broad hall of the temple in Coptos from the archive of this goddess, which this land was in darkness and it was Thoth who shone on this book on all its way," and this book was brought as a valuable treasure to King Khufu of the 4th Dynasty of the Old Kingdom. The significance of this text lies in the fact that it mentions the re-discovery of an already old and forgotten medical text indicating that it originated before the time of Khufu. A further indication of the later date of the compilation is also found in two texts of the London papyrus (Lo.44, 51) which state that these remedies were perfected in the days of King Amenophis III of the 18th Dynasty.

Occasionally, the geographical origins of the contents are indicated in the texts. In the Ebers papyrus a herbal remedy (Eb.188) is simply noted as being made by a physician, but in another passage (Eb.419), a prescription is mentioned as being invented by a high priest of Heliopolis Khui, pointing to Heliopolitan origin. An indication of foreign origin is found where an eye remedy is referred to as being imparted by an Asiatic from Byblos (Eb.422). Additionally, foreign influences on Egyptian medicine are confirmed by the inclusion of seven foreign incantations in the London papyrus (Lo.27–33). Six of these incantations are written in Northwest Semitic dialects and one in the language of Crete, transcribed into syllabic Egyptian script.[155] Ritner (2000: 110) notes, "These prescriptions are in no way marginalized in the papyrus manuscript but fall within a series of typically Egyptian recipes as fully legitimate remedies. Several of the incantations also contain Egyptian passages inserted meaningfully within the larger Semitic text. These interpolated phrases and the proper use of word dividers (determinatives) in Semitic sections show that the scribe actually understood the foreign text and adapted it for his Egyptian audience." The Hearst papyrus (He.170)

[154] Meulenbeld (1987: 2) notes "Clues pointing to the heterodoxy of old medical traditions are still found in the extant versions of the classical *Samhitās*."

[155] For detail, see Steiner (1992).

also includes an incantation against "Semitic disease."[156] A medicinal substance, the *gngnt*-plant, is explained as "like Cretan beans" in the Ebers papyrus (Eb.28).

The Ebers and Hearst papyri (Eb.242–7; He.71–5) contain six prescriptions where claim is made that they were made by the deities Ra, Shu, Tefnut, Geb, Nut and Isis. These prescriptions do not appear to be different from other remedies, and this indication of the divine origin of the remedies is often thought to be a mere assertion of the older origin and sacredness of the remedy (see p. 89–90).

These types of evidence clearly indicate that the Egyptian medical papyri consist of many texts of different temporal and geographical origin; and from this we can conclude that the ancient Egyptian physicians, just like physicians of other cultures (see p. 18), meticulously gathered earlier medical texts, copying and compiling them into new papyri; thus the medical texts were preserved and transmitted throughout a long medical tradition. In fact, the textual transmission of the medical knowledge is mentioned in a text in the paragraph on the ricinus-plant (Eb.251) which states that is according to what is found in the old writings (see p. 28). The medical papyri also exhibit signs of repeated copying activities. One such sign are the many overlaps which occur among the medical papyri. Several texts appear in the same wording or in slightly modified form (e.g. Eb.1 = He.78; Eb.4–6 = He.53, 55, 56; Eb.55 = Bln.2; Eb.122 = Bln.35; Eb.487 = Lo.51; Eb.49 = Lo.17), and also there is a group of paragraphs similarly duplicated (e.g. Eb.221–6 = He.79–84; Eb.277–80 = He.63–6; Eb.499–500 = Lo.47–8; Eb.714–5 = Sm.verso. XXI, 3–8). Duplications may even occur within a papyrus, probably by mistake, as in the Ebers papyrus a few passages are repeated with only slight variations (e.g. Eb.102 = Eb.296; Eb.191–2 = Eb.194–5; Eb.276 = Eb.281). At times the same prescriptions are repeated in different places (e.g. Eb.132–7 = Eb.147–52). These duplications suggest that the contents of the medical papyri are commonly known and important enough to be reproduced as well as passed on.

It should also be noted that although there is no particular paragraph in the Kahun papyrus that has an exact parallel text in other papyri, there is considerable similarity in content (e.g. Kh.21 & RaIV C; Kh.26 & Bln.196; Kh.27 & Bln.193; Kh.28 & Car.IV), and this may indicate that the medicine could have been transmitted by ways other than copying the text.

Another sign of the careful preservation and transmission of the medical texts is the term *gm wš* ("found destroyed") which occasionally appears written in red ink in the middle of the texts (e.g. Eb.57, 738, 755). It does not make any grammatical and contextual sense in the text; and it can be reasonably assumed that while the scribe was copying he found some parts of an original text, which itself could have been a third or fourth copy of an older work, which was damaged and unreadable, and he simply noted that it was unreadable (see p. 60).

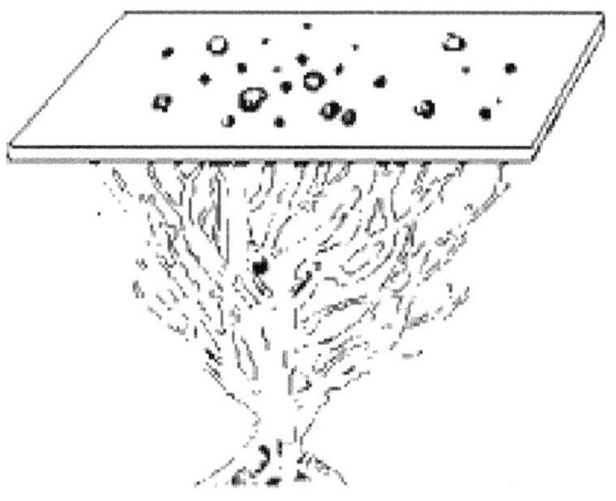

Fig. 8: Tree metaphor: a text/prescription which is reproduced through copying is expressed by ramifying branches.

In addition, the glosses, which are occasionally attached to the main text and provide an explanation of the meaning of a word or statement that appears in the main text, also reflect the transmission of the text. We can assume that such glosses were added by someone who worked on the text in succession to help others to understand it. Sometimes we even find a gloss attached to a previous gloss (see p. 36, 61).

The philological study of Egyptian medical papyri can also reveal the older origin of their contents. In most cases the grammatical structure of medical texts points to a date in the Middle Kingdom, but some scholars have remarked that the language of particular texts is particularly archaic and shows peculiarities not encountered after the Old Kingdom.[157] The clearest feature revealing the diversity in the origin of the texts is the orthographical variation, particularly of material names. These are found throughout the papyri. Weeks (1976–78: 294–5) provides several examples from the Ebers papyrus: the word *nkʿwt*, which usually translates as "notched sycamore fruit," occurs twenty-five times and exhibits three different spellings. The unidentified plant material *sht* occurs eight times and shows five variant spelling, and only two of these writings occur more than once. The substance *prt-šny*, a kind of plant, occurs forty-three times and shows seven variant spellings. And he notes that in some cases as many as twenty different spellings of a single material name occur and are widely distributed throughout the papyri.

156 This spell is written in Egyptian language and includes Egyptian gods.

157 Kurt Sethe's assertion is quoted by Sigerist (1951: 299); Nunn (1996: 27) notes "Both Breasted (1930) and Westendorf (1992) have expressed the view that the original must have been Old Kingdom on the grounds of some items of grammatical construction and vocabulary. This would be about 1000 years before the copy we possess. However, most of the text is written in classical Middle Egyptian and the early origin of the papyrus has recently been questioned by Collin, Parkinson and Quirke (personal communications, 1995). It would not be unusual if certain archaic features had been deliberately introduced into the text to give the appearance of antiquity, which was so revered by the ancient Egyptian."

Weeks (1976–78) considers that these orthographical variations of material names in the Ebers papyrus not randomly distributed, and he claims that with the studying the occurrence of orthographical variations, it would be possible to extract clusters of texts which may be distinguished as the sources from which the Ebers papyrus is compiled. Weeks (1976–78: 295) gives a description of the arrangement of the Ebers papyrus: prescription groups are defined by their subject-matter, and the groups are clearly marked by the occurrence of phrases such as "The Beginning of Treatments for …" preceding a group of prescriptions. Weeks also observes that the orthographic variants distribute themselves in near-perfect correlation with these prescription groups (see p. 77). After further considerations, he concludes that this orthographic analysis suggests the Ebers papyrus had as its source twenty-five to thirty earlier papyri (Weeks 1976–78: 295).[158]

5.2 Medical papyri and physicians' activity

In general, we are unable to ascertain the precise function and role of the medical papyrus in ancient Egypt. The medial papyrus might have been a collection kept in a temple library as a reference work, or in a diagnostic text, a textual expression such as "if you examine …" or "you shall say concerning him …" may indicate that the papyrus was a teaching book for students of medicine. On the other hand, the papyrus may have been used in actual practice by physicians in their treatment. Sometimes the Ebers and Edwin Smith papyri are thought to have been funerary objects because they are both mentioned as having been found in a tomb near Luxor.[159] This view is supported by the good state of preservation of these papyri. Overall, the general nature of the medical writings is a very practical one, and even in the Ebers papyrus we find signs of the actual use of this papyrus, as Joachim (1890)[160] describes:

> The papyrus has undoubtedly been used; slight inaccuracies in the text have been corrected, consequent, I believe, on its use—sometimes, indeed, with paler ink than that in which the papyrus is written, as one can clearly make out. On the margin of the page there are now and then short remarks; for instance—probably by a later user—on the margin of page 40 the word nefr = 'good' has been added three times in pale ink, different from the original; on page 41 there are on the margin the words nefr ar = 'good to prepare'

Maspéro (1909: 269) comments that "one of the owners of the Ebers papyrus had occasion to try several of his most advantageous prescriptions on his patient, and when they were successful he wrote *good* on the margin by each, for the instruction of his successors and the edification of posterity."

In one prescription (Eb.509) we find the note added "really effective. I have seen (it). It has often happened to me," and elsewhere (Eb.356) "Do this, you will see (the success)." Such notes indicating the efficacy of prescriptions occur frequently (e.g. Eb.351, 386, 636, 648), and at times such notes can occur in the middle of a prescription (e.g. Eb.356, 636), inferring that they are copies of previous notes. A comment "really effective many times" (e.g. Eb.386), which is often found, may indicate that the copier found "good" marked several times on the prescription by several physicians through the succession of the papyrus, and he may have used this comment as a generic expression of this fact. The continuation of the custom of marking recommendations of successful prescriptions for later users is showed in the Coptic medical papyrus in words such as "we have experimented with this remedy and found it perfect" (Chas.26), "I have experienced with (this powder) and found it perfect, it is without equal in efficacy" (Chas.109), and "a powder experimented upon by ourselves. We have tried it and have found it useful for all maladies of the eyes" (Chas.80) (Chassinat 1921: 109, 130, 190; Dawson 1923–24: 56).[161]

A marl clay cup dated roughly to the fifth or fourth century BC[162] may carry evidence for a treatment by the way of a prescription from the medical papyrus. The cup is inscribed in hieratic with the words *tpnn smi bit* ("cumin, set milk, honey") in black ink. Poole (2001: 175) found that the same recipe for a cough appears in the Berlin papyrus (Bln.31, 47) and some similar recipes in this section for the treatment of a cough (Bln.29–47)[163] include two of these three substances (*smi* and *bit* in Bln.29 = Eb.315, Bln.34; *smi* and *tpnn* in Bln.41). Poole (2001: 179–80) provides a comment:

> The Naples cup is one of the few surviving examples of a labelled ancient Egyptian medicine container. It is also, to my knowledge, the only one inscribed with a

[158] Such clusters of original texts may have consisted of earlier writings.

[159] These two papyri were purchased by Edwin Smith in 1862 from a local merchant in Luxor, but by the time the importance of the papyri was recognised the finder had already died, and the tomb from which these papyri were taken has never been identified. The papyri seem to have remained in his possession until at least 1869 when they appeared in a catalogue of antiquities. Both were originally known as the Papyrus Smith until 1873. But one part appeared as the Ebers papyrus in a publication by George Ebers in 1873. In 1875, Ebers published a superb facsimile edition with Egyptian-Latin vocabulary and introduction. In it he noted that in the winter of 1872–73, while in Thebes, he was offered this papyrus by a resident there. He was informed that it had been obtained fourteen years earlier from a grave at El Assassif and had been found between the legs of a mummy (Comrie 1909: 120; Nunn 1996: 25–30); See also Klein (1905: 1929).

[160] Comrie's (1909: 120) quote of Joachim's note in "Papyrus Ebers, das älteste Buch über Heilkunde, aus dem Aegyptischen zum erstenmal vollständig übersetzt."

[161] In her ethnographic study of contemporary Egypt, Blackman (1927, reprinted in 2000: 207, 311) notes her finding close parallels with the Ebers papyrus in appended comments such as "Tried and true" in prescriptions used by a Sheikh, a medicine-man, in a village of Upper Egypt.

[162] This clay cup is now preserved in the National Archaeological Museum of Naples (inv. no. 828).

[163] With the exception of prescription Bln.35 (= Eb.122) which is designated as a treatment against *wḥdw*.

remedy listed in the medical papyri. This is all the more remarkable because of the wide chronological gap between the cup and the Berlin papyrus. The former dates from the fifth to fourth century BC, the latter from the Nineteenth Dynasty. Thus the recipe must have been handed down for some 700 years at the very least, and probably many more, since the medical lore compiled in the Berlin papyrus must be much older.

We may, therefore, assume that the prescriptions recorded in the medical papyri were frequently used for reference and remedies were prepared according to the prescription by the physicians, and thus a medical papyrus may well have been an essential item for the physicians.[164] Whatever we may speculate, the actual situation and the activities of Egyptian physicians are quite unknown.

Physicians' duty in the medical institution

The institution called *prw ʿnḫ* (lit. "House of Life") which was attached to temples is generally considered the centre of medical activities in ancient Egypt. The chief *prw ʿnḫ* so far known were in Memphis, Saïs, Heliopolis, Thebes, Abydos, Amarna, Akhmim, Coptos, Esna, Edfu and Bubastis, and archaeological evidence suggests that the *prw ʿnḫ* at Saïs flourished as early as the Third Dynasty (Gordon and Schwabe 2004: 154–62). Sometimes it has been suggested that the *prw ʿnḫ* functioned as medical schools, providing medical education and training to young physicians, but in fact, its precise function is not known.[165] The practice of medical research in ancient Egypt is inferred from the writing of Africanus and Eusebius, quoting the lost works of the Egyptian historian Manetho. Africanus wrote: "Athothis, his (i.e. Menes') son, for 57 years. He built the palace at Memphis; and his anatomical works are extent, for he was a physician" (trans. Waddell 1940: 29).[166] Nunn (1996: 42) comments:

> Although the citation of Manetho is consistent, no systematic Egyptian work on anatomy has survived, and it is very difficult to believe that there was any serious study of anatomy at the beginning of the third millennium BC. It is almost certain that no appropriate climate of enquiry existed at that time. Nevertheless, the anatomical insight shown for certain parts of the body in some of the medical papyri, the Edwin Smith in particular, strongly supports the view that there had been quite detailed study of anatomy at an early date and it is possible that a treatise on anatomy might have existed.

Some 150 Egyptian physicians, ranging from the Third Dynasty to the Twenty-seventh Dynasty, are known to us.[167] The titles held by these physicians are gleaned from stelae and wall-reliefs in their tombs or those of their patrons, and these titles introduce some broader ideas concerning aspects of the physicians' activities. There are several kinds of title, that are noticeably attributed to the physicians. The titles such as *wr swnw m st mȝʿt* ("chief physician in the Place of Truth" [the necropolis]) and *swnw sȝ* ("physician of the troop")[168] may provide some ideas about the environment of the physicians' activity. The physicians' royal connections are indicated through the titles such as *swnw pr ʿȝ* ("physician of the palace"), *swnw n nsw* ("physician to the king"), *swnw n pr ḥmt nsw* ("physician to the house of the queen") and *swnw n nb tȝwy* ("physician to the Lord of the Two Land").[169] The significant feature of the physician's title

[164] Harris (1971: 115) notes Horapollo's statement that the Egyptian physicians possessed a book called *ambrēs*, from which they were able to predetermine the outcome of an illness. Nunn (1996: 131) comments "there can be little doubt that the medical papyri fulfilled a role no less important than that of medical texts today. Many were in a format which simply listed remedies for named diseases, and these were clearly intended for reference because the drugs available to the ancient Egyptians were far too numerous to remember"; Stephan (1997) argues that the medical texts are not just case studies but that they also indicate texts used in "academic" instruction. He concludes that one can detect aprioristic (patho-) physiological concepts that are only conceivable in the context of organised forms of instruction (Stephan 1997: 301).

[165] This view is largely based on an inscribed statue of the physician *Wedja-hor-resnet* (Vatican Museum, 22690), in which he recorded that Darius (the second king of the 27th (Persian) Dynasty) commanded him "to restore the department(s) of the house(s) of life (dealing with medicine) after (they had fallen into) decay," and *Wedja-hor-resnet* "placed them in the charge of every learned man (in order to teach them?) their craft(s) … this his majesty did because he knew the virtue of this art to revive all that are sick …" (Gardiner 1938: 157; Nunn 1996: 131; Westendorf 1999: 476; Stephan 2005: 86); Comrie (1909: 112) notes that Josephus (*Contra Apionem*, I, 26) quotes the statement of Manetho, that Moses was a priest at Heliopolis, a great medical centre of his time, and these physicians received their preliminary training in the temples; Some scholars consider the physicians received their training in the *pr ʿnḫ*, suggesting the it might have been something analogous to the modern medical school and those of Greece and Alexandria, but others assert this view is unlikely (Gardiner 1938: 159). Weber (1980: 954) states that the House of Life was an "Institution, in der wissenschaftliche und religiöse Werke der alten Ägypter verfaßt, kopiert und aufbewahrt wurden und wo durch ein eigenes Ritual für die Erhaltung des Lebens in der Welt gesorgt wurde … Seit Gardiner's Arbeit wird das L. (Lebenshaus) häufig überspitzt als eine Art scriptorium beschrieben oder gar noch allgemeiner als 'Universität.' Doch war das L. vor allem ein für das Land zentraler Kultplatz"; Meulenaere (1975: 80) also mentions "Il est peu probable qu'on y offrait un enseignement scientifique organise"; Nunn (1996: 131) assumes "it is likely that master copies would be preserved in the *per ʿnḫ*, and fortunate doctors would have their own copies; Ghalioungui (1973: 66) notes "Large collections of books were kept in these houses (*per ankh*) even as late as the 3rd century A.D. when Galen wrote that physicians still visited the library of the school of Memphis (Galen, *de composit. Medicament*, V, 2)."

[166] Eusebius' version of Manetho reads "Athothis, his son, ruled for 27 years. He built the palace at Memphis; he practiced medicine and wrote anatomical books" (trans. Waddell 1940: 31); Westendorf (1992: 40) questions whether one can take Manetho's statement literally: "Nun gehört es zur Geschichtsschreibung, daß den ersten Königen generell alles zugeordnet wird, was es an einschneidenden Neuerungen gab: sie fungierten gleichsam als Kultur-Heroen. Auf diesem Hintergrunde müssen wir auch diese Nachricht sehen, von der wir aber auch objektiv sagen dürfen, das sie so nicht stimmen kann."

[167] For a concise summary of known Egyptian physicians, see Jonckheere (1951; 1958), Habachi *et al.* (1969–70) and Ghalioungui (1983: 16–37); Ghalioungui (1983: 38–50) and Nunn (1996: 116–29) provide useful summaries on the titles of Egyptian physicians.

[168] These translations are based on Jonckeere's translation (1958: 38, 79) "Chef des médecins de la Place de Vérité (Nécroploe)" and "Médecin de la troupe."

[169] 39 of 150 physicians displayed royal connections, and it is likely that the list of 150 physicians is heavily biased in favour of those in an exalted position, who were in a "goodly burial," which ensured that their memory survived.

is that it includes an indication of medical specialisation. We find titles like *swnw ẖt* ("physician of the abdomen"), which can be interpreted as meaning gastro-enterologist and *swnw irty* ("physician of the eyes") which may mean ophthalmologist. Other obscure titles which physicians carry are *ibḥ* ("teeth") which may be understood as dentist[170] and *nr pḥwyt* (lit. "herdsman of the anus") which may be considered as proctologist.[171] A more obscure title is *swnw ꜣꜥꜥ mw m ḥnw nṯnṯ.t*, which can be translated as "physician interpreter of the liquids hidden in the *nṯnṯ.t*" (Westendorf 1999: 475)[172] and *swnw ꜣꜥꜥ ḥm(w).t štꜣ.t*, which is "physician interpreter of the secret art" (Ghalioungui 1983: 43).[173] There is no known Egyptian word for "veterinary" other than the epithet *rḫ kꜣw* (lit. "one who knows the bulls") (Ghalioungui 1983: 12–3; Nunn 1996: 120), but the expertise of the veterinary in Egypt is seen in the Veterinary Papyrus of Kahun.[174] These indications of medical specialisation in ancient Egypt remind us of a statement by Herodotus (II, 84) that "medicine is practiced among Egyptians on a plane of separation; each physician is a physician of one disease and no more; thus the whole country is full of physicians, for some profess themselves to be physicians of the eyes, others of the head, others of the teeth, others of the affections of intestines, and some those which are not local" (trans. Macaulay 1904: 152). This record of Egyptian medical specialisation attested in the Greek period accords well with the titles of pharaonic physicians. Another type of physician's title is one that relates to the hierarchical bureaucratic administration of the medical institution, such as *ḫrp swnw* ("administrator of physicians"), *ḥry swnw* and *imy-rꜣ swnw* ("overseer of physicians"), *sḥḏ swwnw* ("inspector of physicians") and *wr swnw* ("chief physician"), and these titles would indicate the Egyptians' establishment of an organised medical institution.[175]

Despite this, it is difficult to assume any aspect of physicians' activities based on the indications of their titles. Grapow (1956: 95) comments on this difficulty saying that ancient Egyptian titles, medical or non-medical alike, are meaningless to us as far as the activities of their holders go, one wonders how truly informative they are (Hussein 1998: 55). This difficulty in comprehending physicians' titles is also noted by Breasted (1930: 171, 543) who warns that there is a danger of confusion arising from the fact that titles indicative of rank or office suffer great changes in meaning in the lapse of several thousand years and that they cannot be determined with precision.

Medical specialization, in the modern sense, derives from the need for physicians to focus professionally on one or two particular areas of expertise owing to the complexity and range of knowledge in the entire field of medicine. Such specialisation requires tailor-made courses of education and training. Sometimes an understanding of ancient Egyptian medical specialisation is made in this sense. Sigerist (1951: 319) comments that "Egyptologists are inclined to assume that as early as the Old Kingdom medical knowledge was so highly developed that the individual physician could no longer embrace it and specialization became unavoidable." The actual significance of the Egyptian specialisation remains obscure.

Similarly, when we think about the meaning of the bureaucratic organisation of medical institutions, we tend to assume that its significance resides in the distribution of authority throughout the institutional system, and each physician is assigned his responsibility, and his activity is regulated and supervised in the organisational system enforced by the state. Concerning the responsibility and the regulations of the Egyptian physicians, some ideas can be derived from the description of the Egyptian physician of the Greek period given by Diodorus Siculus (I, 82):

> for the physicians draw their support from public funds and administer their treatments in accordance with a written law which was composed in ancient times by many famous physicians. If they follow the rules of this law as they read them in the sacred book and yet are unable to save their patient, they are absolved and go unpunished; but if they go contrary to the law's prescriptions in any respect, they must submit to a trial with death as the penalty, the lawgiver holding that but few physicians would ever show themselves wiser than the mode of treatment which had been closely followed for a long period and had been originally prescribed by the ablest physician (trans. Oldfather 1933: 281).

Aristotle (*Politics,* 3.15) also mentions the regulation governing Egyptian physician of his time, stating that he was allowed to alter the treatment prescribed by authority after the fourth day but if he did so before this he bore the risk.[176] Nothing of the law of pharaonic Egypt governing the physicians has survived.[177] But the assigning of responsibility to physicians' activities and the setting up of regulations and punishment seem to be common practice in the civilized cultures of antiquity. There is a well-known contemporary medical law in the Codex of Hammurabi

[170] There has been much dispute concerning the identification as dentist; see, for example, the discussions in Leek (1969, 1972) and Ghalioungui (1971).

[171] Ghalioungui (1983: 7) assumes this title may be comparable to the Greek *iatrokleiston*, "enema dispenser."

[172] The word *nṯnṯ.t* cannot at present be translated; See Hussein (1998) and Westendorf (1999: 475, n.9); Stephan (2005: 82) notes "Dazu kamen wohl Helfer wie Krankenpfleger, Assistenten, Masseure und Therapeuten."

[173] Hussein (2001: 29) suggests that the title *swnw ꜣꜥꜥ ḥm(w).t štꜣ.t* can be understood as "physician who interpret the secret acts concerning sex" and notes that this job is still practiced in upper Egypt.

[174] On the Veterinary Papyrus of Kahun, see Froehner (1934) and Walker (1964).

[175] On the hierarchical administration and specialisation of Egyptian physicians indicated by their title, see also Westendorf (1999: 472–5).

[176] Translation by Barker (1946: 141) is "In Egypt it is permissible for doctors to alter the rules of treatment after the first four days, though a doctor who alters them earlier does so at his own risk."

[177] Aristotle (*Politics*, 7.10) mentions "The history of Egypt attests the antiquity of all political institutions. The Egyptians are generally accounted the oldest people on earth; and they have always had a body of law and a system of politics" (trans. Barker 1946: 304).

that states, for instance, "if a physician has made a deep incision with a surgeon's knife on a man and has saved the man's life, or has opened out a man's eye-socket and saved the man's sight, he shall receive ten shekels of silver … if a physician has made a deep incision with a surgeon's knife on a man and has caused the man's death, or has opened out a man's eye-socket and destroyed the man's sight, they shall cut off his hand" (L.215–18; trans. Richardson 2004: 107). Comparable regulation and punishment can be found in China and India.[178] The duty of the physician and medical ethics in Greece is clearly reflected in the famous Hippocratic Oath, which reads: "I swear by Apollo Physician and Asclepius and Hygieia and Panaceia and all the gods and goddesses … I will apply dietic measures for the benefit of the sick according to my ability and judgment; I will keep them from harm and injustice. I will neither give a deadly drug to anybody if asked for it, nor will I make a suggestion to this effect … If I fulfil this oath and do not violate it, may it be granted to me enjoy life and art, being honoured with fame among all men for all time to come; if I transgress it and swear falsely, may the opposite of all this be my lot" (Temkin *et al.* 1967: 6).[179] Evidence of ancient medical ethics based on a difficult text in the Ebers papyrus (Eb.205, 206) is sometimes suggested *ꜥḳ r-f m bṯ sw* which Ebbell (1937: 53–4) translates "Go in to him and do not abandon him!"[180]

5.3 Traditionalism in Egyptian medicine

Standard format of medical text

Although the precise significance of the early specialisation of medicine and bureaucratic medical organisation is not clear, the observations outlined above may point to a situation that the Egyptians had already achieved the formulation of a well-established medical tradition by the early stages of the Dynastic Period. In the medical papyri, we can find several features that point toward such an established medical tradition of ancient Egypt. One such feature is the relative consistency of textual format throughout the papyri. In diagnostic texts we find a stock format, always referring to the reader as "you" and speaking of the patient as "man," "woman" or "one who is suffering from …" The texts of the Kahun papyrus, the oldest preserved papyrus, have a slightly different expression, but still follow this standard format. The prognostic texts, which are regularly instructed to be stated by a physician in the Edwin Smith papyrus and in some instances in other papyri (e.g. Eb.857–62), show three cases using stock phrases "an ailment which I will treat", "an ailment which I will contend" and "an ailment not to be treated." Also in the Edwin Smith papyrus, apart from flesh wounds and dislocations, all injuries fall into three categories: *sd* ("smashing"), *pšn* ("splitting") or *thm* ("piercing") (Iversen 1953: 164).[181] There also appears to have been a standard for the length of treatment as in most of the prescriptions in medical papyri, the treatment is instructed to be 4 days (see p. 60).

Practical arrangement of medical texts

One can recognise an attempt at establishing a classification of clinical matter in the medical papyri (see p. 23-4). The Kahun, Carlsberg and Ramesseum papyri, for instance, are characterised by the treatment of ailments of women and gynaecological matters, the Chester Beatty papyrus (VI) concentrates on rectal diseases, the Edwin Smith papyrus deals with surgical treatment, while the Ebers, Hearst, Berlin and London papyri mainly provide prescriptions for internal and external ailments (Westendorf 1999: 545). The classification of clinical matters is also apparent in the arrangement of the Ebers papyrus, which, as the largest papyrus, contains many prescriptions for many kinds of ailments (see p. 75-6). The clinical matters in the Ebers papyrus are roughly classified according to diseases of the abdomen, of the skin, rectal ailments, urinary problems, eye diseases, diseases of woman, wounds and injuries, as well as statements of anatomo-physiological knowledge and some miscellaneous records. An unusual aspect of the Ebers papyrus is the numbering of pages noted at the top of each column up to 110 pages.[182] This marking of pages may be due to the considerable size of this papyrus making it necessary to provide page numbers so that the user could easily find the section he wished to refer to.

---

178 In India, for instance, the *Arthasastra* (iv.1) prescribes a fine if a patient dies while receiving medical attention and the authorities are not informed, and a heavier one if his death is brought about by neglect or inadequate medical knowledge on the part of the doctor. A lesser fine is prescribed for permanent injury caused by bad treatment (Basham 1976: 33).

179 Temkin *et al.* (1967: 63) states "As time went on, the Hippocratic Oath became the nucleus of all medical ethics. In all countries, in all epochs in which monotheism, in its purely religious or in its more secularised form, was the accepted creed, the Hippocratic Oath was applauded as the embodiment of truth. Not only Jews and Christians, but the Arabs, the mediaeval doctors, men of the Renaissance, scientists of the Enlightenment, and scholars of the nineteenth century embraced the ideals of the Oath."

180 Ghalioungui (1987: 68–9) translates this text "go against it (the disease). Do not go out of its way," and provides a comment that "The description of the case is in general and in particular full of contradictions: first, a refusal of treatment; then a fight with the disease and, in conclusion, one should go on against it. Is it a description of a stepwise improvement?"; The requirement of the physician to fulfil his ethical duty is also seen in a text: "you shall not be remiss therewith" (Eb.710).

181 Iversen (1953: 163–9) observes, from the comparative study of the types of injury identified in the Edwin Smith papyrus and the Hippocratic corpus (*On Wounds in the Head*), that "Not only have both sides arrived at three intrinsically well-defined basic types, of which all other lesions are regarded as variants, but the Greek and the Egyptian conceptions of the Characters of these basic types clearly coincide." The correspondent injuries of Egyptian and Greek are *sd* and φλάσις, *pšn* and ῥῆγμα, and *thm* and ἕδρα (Iversen 1953: 168–9); Ghalioungui (1973: 43) notes "Harris points out that in comparable Hippocratic works there are again three types of injury … that may be shown to correspond closely to the Egyptian classification. Harris concludes that, apart from trephining, the Hippocratic Corpus may be seen to follow closely Egyptian medical tradition …"

182 This papyrus has 108 columns, but the scribe wrongly numbered them, giving the number 110 the last column, and columns 28 and 29 were dropped out for unknown reasons (Ghalioungui 1987: 3).

Another example of a practical arrangement for reference purposes is found in the Edwin Smith papyrus, in which the forty-eight cases of trauma it contains are arranged from the head down through the body.[183]

Conservative practice of traditional medicine

Scholars tend to assume that the establishment of Egyptian medicine and medical tradition took place in relatively early times, and at least by the time our papyri were composed, the contents of medical papyri were already traditional and authoritative, and as noted in the statements by Diodorus and Aristotle, for example, Egyptian physicians of their time were using treatments prescribed by an ancient authority recorded in a sacred book and they were not allowed to render their own treatments unless they accept responsibility for their outcomes; this means pharaonic physicians had to follow the treatment methods recorded in their traditional medical papyri. Concerning the time at which this Egyptian achievement occurred, Grapow concludes from the linguistic features of diagnosis that are analogous those to of mechanical texts, in conjunction with the fact that the designations of drugs do not contain new words, that ancient Egyptian medicine reached its full development and maturity before 1600 BC; and in the time of the New Kingdom it degenerated into sorcery (quoted from Leake 1940: 316). So we may believe, as Aristotle notes, that physicians were allowed to alter the treatment prescribed by authority after the forth day, four days being the duration of the application of treatment which Egyptian prescriptions mostly instruct and which may also have been a standard period after which a remedy could be altered.[184] Concerning the selection and altering of prescriptions by physicians, Weeks (1976–78: 296) notes an important feature showed in the Ebers papyrus namely that the first prescriptions in any prescription group are generally short ones, containing only three or four materials and administered in relatively small dosages. Prescriptions further down the list tend to contain more materials and increased dosages. The last prescriptions in a group are usually the longest. He also notes that the final prescriptions tend to include references to religious acts or incantations to be performed and recited. For Weeks this ordering points toward a procedure in the treatment of a patient whereby the Egyptian physician would have begun his treatment with small doses of a few drugs from the early prescriptions in a group, and then if need be administered larger doses and more complex prescriptions, with the religious treatments as the final option after all the other remedies have been tried out (Weeks 1976–78: 296) (see p. 77).

The conservative traditionalism of ancient Egyptian culture is often pointed to as the reason for the physician's faithful adherence to old traditional medicine. Ritner (2000: 107) states that "Typically, ancient Egypt has been viewed as a quintessentially conservative culture, dedicated to the preservation of traditional concepts and techniques scrupulously maintained through the centuries with little or no modification. In the Ptolemaic era, the Greek historian Diodorus Siculus even records legislative penalties for methodological innovation by state-supported physicians in the army." Furthermore, Nunn (1996: 206) observes "There is no evidence of major changes in the format or content of classical Egyptian medicine between the Old Kingdom and the end of the Twenty-Sixth Dynasty, covering the years 2600 to 525 BC. This may be ascribed to the innate conservatism of the Egyptians, their geographical isolation and their relative freedom from foreign domination." We can see from the extent of duplication of the same or similar texts found among the papyri dating to different times that traditional medicine was conservatively preserved and repeatedly practiced with a minimum of modification.[185] In addition, the Egyptian's particular faithfulness to their medical tradition is reflected in the variation of spellings that Weeks (1976–78: 294) points out "The (standard) orthography of the early Eighteenth Dynasty—and we know that Papyrus Ebers was written in the ninth year of the reign of Amenhotep I, about 1537 B.C., certain recent questions of this fact notwithstanding—the orthography of the early Eighteenth Dynasty showed a uniform and regular pattern. Drug names in P. Ebers, however, are spelled in a number of different ways, and in some cases as many as twenty different spellings of a single drug name occur." We may also judge from the note "found destroyed" marked by Egyptian copiers that no guessing was allowed in filling in a missing part. Thus, it can be assumed there was a consistent mode of therapy based on established traditional medical ideas in ancient Egypt throughout the Dynastic Period. Ritner (2000: 107) states:

> The claim of extraordinary antiquity for this book was certainly not intended to indicate its obsolescence but, rather, to bolster its authority and presumed validity. 'Progress' is a notion alien to Egypt and most ancient cultures, which view the current and future ages as 'regressions' from an ideal 'Golden Age' when

[183] The extant copy of this papyrus stops abruptly in the middle of Case 48, in the middle of a sentence and shortly after the scribe dipped his pen in the ink and retraced the last two signs he had written (Nunn 1996: 29). If this papyrus had been intended to continue down to the toe, it would have been a massive papyrus when completed: the arrangement of the ailments according to individual body parts in the top-to-toe sequence is the customary arrangement found in many cultures (Dawson 1932–33: 36); King (2001: 6) notes that the medical work from Mesopotamia known as *The Diagnostic Handbook* forms a "head to foot" arrangement of detailed observations of symptoms.

[184] Halioua *et al.* (2005: 87) states "Medicines were not prescribed for longer than four days, perhaps a symbolic period of time given that the number four was considered, particularly during the Old Kingdom, to have magical and beneficial value."

[185] The root of Egyptian conservative traditionalism may be seen in their notion of *sp-tpy* or "First Occasion," the moment the creator god emerged and the universe was set out in order. Egyptians often refer to a situation which is "like the First Occasion," for the repetitions of the First Occasion assure continuity of the world. Significance of repetitions of old tradition is also seen in practicing of *sni r* ("imitate") (Faulkner 1962: 230); On the *sp-tpy*, see Gundlach (1986) and Dunand (2004: 52–5); For examples of the Egyptian use of *sni*, see Ockinga (1983: 93–4).

mankind and divinity more closely interacted. In Egypt, the notion of an ideal past is linked to complex philosophical understandings of time itself, viewed as a repeating cycle or spiral capable of being manipulated by ritual. On a theoretical level, 'progress' was neither desirable nor necessary. Situations, individuals, and techniques were said to be improved (*snfr*), but such improvement is almost invariably termed a 're-creation' of prior favourable conditions. Thus restorative ritual and medicine 'renewed' or 'rejuvenated' by returning the individual to an ideal former state and time.

Ritner then comments that the glosses attached to the original texts were actually modernizations of the older texts.

Oral transmission of the secret of medicine

When forming an understanding of ancient Egyptian traditionalism and its manner of preserving a consistent mode of medical theory, it is apposite to refer to Sivin's (1995) comparative study of Greek and Chinese cultures. In his work, Sivin (1995: 8) describes the differences between these two cultures, whereby the Greeks, who depended on skill in debate for their livelihood and fame, tended to argue face to face and to expect the public to decide, just as it decided in the assembly or at trials. In contrast, the Chinese, who lived by their knowledge, usually presented their ideas not to colleagues but rather to their patrons, who expected advice but did not have to act on it, or even to reply to it. Consequently for them, disagreements with other scholars were unimportant. Sivin then summarises that Greek culture encouraged disagreement and disputation in natural philosophy and science as in every other field since oral disagreement was a tool of competition, while in China the emphasis remained on consensus. I think, in this respect, Egyptian culture was possibly closer to Chinese practices rather than the Greek style. The characteristics of Greek culture described by Sivin are evident in the Greek medical papyri. For instance, the Hippocratic corpus, which consists of sixty treatises varying in subject matter and style, includes some texts which appear to be public lectures since they are written in the first person and often seem dogmatic, arguing a point. An author could discuss his own individual ideas and could even criticise other ways of thinking. Other sections of writing may arise from teachings as they resemble lecture notes, or even take the form of a simple sentence summarising particular situations. Such a writing style is entirely absent in ancient Egyptian literature. The Egyptian mathematical papyri provide examples for practice but do not provide any explanation for the mathematical formulae or equations.[186] Likewise, Egyptian myths can describe the roles of divinities and the structure of the universe in the form of a tale but they do not directly mention a theological principle.[187] Likewise, the medical papyri all provide cases of treatments and not a medical theory. It seems the Egyptians were either intentionally concealing the important parts of their knowledge from their writings or disclosure of medical knowledge was restricted.[188]

The restriction of medical knowledge is nearly universal in antiquity. This also applies in ancient Greece as evidenced in the Hippocratic Oath, which includes the undertaking "to give a share of precepts and oral instruction and all the other learning to my sons and to the sons of him who has instructed me and to pupils who have signed the covenant and have taken an oath according to medical law, but to no one else" (Temkin 1967: 6). Nonetheless, the Greek physician, having been accepted to learn medicine, could produce explicit texts, while strict observance of the restrictions on passing on medical knowledge is made clear by the word "secret" which occasionally appears in the Egyptian medical texts.[189] Instructions to keep the medicine secret in the Ebers papyrus (Eb.206) is expressed by the words, "you should then prepare a remedy that is a secret for any relation of the physician, except for your own daughter,"[190] and in the Chester Beatty (VIIm Rs 7,7), "Guard the scroll. Do not permit another to unroll it," "it is a genuine secret; the profane mob dare not know it" and "do not pronounce it to anyone; take care of it all times" (Schwabe 1986: 152; Gordon *et al.* 2004: 187–8).

Thus in ancient Egypt, medical practice throughout the period was largely based on the old and established medical tradition. Important theoretical parts and principles of authoritative and secret medicine were conservatively preserved and transmitted orally over successive generations.[191] We may then conclude that the secret

[186] For general information about the content of Egyptian mathematical papyri, see Chace (1929).

[187] On the lack of canonization in ancient Egypt, Christiane states "Far from wanting to limit their theological reflection by stopping it once and for all and by declaring it untouchable and dogmatic, they preferred to keep their texts open to reflection according to their methods of association and accumulation; it was as though their approach to the divine drew ever greater strength from the multiplication of combinations, borrowing here and there to unite and compare the multiplicity of viewpoints. The Egyptians were fond of glossing" (Dunand *et al.* 2004: xii).

[188] Weber (1980: 955) states "Im L. (Lebenshaus) wird alles 'geheime' Wissen verwahrt. Es existiert dort als eine besondere Abteilung eine Art von Ärzteschule. Ihre Verbundenheit mit dem L. wird u.a. dadurch deulich, daß Ärzte im 6. Jh. v. Chr. die L. von Abydos und Sais restaurierten ... der innere Zusammenhang ist darin zu sehen, daß ja gerade die Ärzte zur Erhaltung des Lebens beitrugen"; On the *prw ꜥnḫ*, see p. 57.

[189] Gordon and Schwabe (2004: 188) compare the secret nature of Egyptian medicine with Spell 161 of the Book of the Dead, which states "No outsider is to know (this spell for) it is secret; the rabble is not to know (it)."

[190] The meaning of "except your own daughter" is difficult to interpret. Ghalioungui (1987: 70) comments: "If our interpretation of this passage is correct, there is possibly here an indication that the secret medical knowledge would be inherited by (the eldest?) daughter. Or is the correct reading *sꜣ.tj* 'male heir',or *zꜣ.t*, 'little son'? "

[191] We may also notice that the medicine is essentially craft that would not be taught and learnt purely by text. Ghalioungui (1973: 51) notes "To take engineering as a point of comparison, no engineer's papyri are known, and few mathematical texts available deal with elementary mathematics. If Egyptian knowledge did not exceed these notions, how could they build a several million ton pyramid with errors of less than an inch and a fraction of a degree, not to speak of the logistic problems the building must have raised. We must, therefore, assume

medical knowledge of medicine was shared only within the society of physicians. But every Egyptian physician learnt the theories and principles of medicine, and could therefore have derived theories and principles even from a very simple text or prescription recorded in the medical papyri. He could then have practiced a form of medicine based on the traditional medical ideas with reference to the old texts, rather than just prescribing remedies according to the text's instructions without knowing the principles that lay behind them. How could they, otherwise, have maintained their fame and reputation throughout history?

5.4 Ebers papyrus: representative of Egyptian medicine?

After all these considerations, when we evaluate the validity of Egyptian medical papyri as bodies for a sample for statistical analysis, there are two possible opposing standpoints. One can assert that the Egyptian papyri are merely a compilation of fragmented texts of different origin, like the medical writings of other cultures; that they comprise a variety of inconsistent medical ideas and that these are combined without taking into account their "Redaktionsgeschichte," i.e. the changes that have probably been made to these texts in a period of perhaps more than a thousand years in the process of textual transmission. All these factors render the validity of the papyri questionable. The other standpoint would emphasise the conservative traditionalism of Egyptian medicine, and assumes that there is consistency in medical theory and practice as well as in the principle of prescription, and that only minimum changes would have been made. The second standpoint would, therefore, regard the papyri as being representative of Egyptian medicine. It is difficult to decide which perspective to support, but if we are to run a statistical analysis, we have to follow the more optimistic second approach.

Nonetheless, we often find assertions of the comprehensive nature of the Ebers papyrus. As early as 1875, Ebers saw his papyrus as "das hermetische Buch über die Arzeneimittel der alten Aegypter in hieratischer Schrift,"[192] because the methods of classifying clinical matters shown in the Ebers papyrus is reminiscent of the lost Hermetic books mentioned by Clement of Alexandria. According to this ancient scholar, the Hermetic books were the sacred books of Thoth kept in the temples during the Greek period (Thissen 1977: 1135–6). They consisted of forty-two books, and thirty-six dealt with philosophy and six with medicine. The latter were texts on the constitution of the body (anatomy), disease, medical instruments (surgery), drugs, diseases of the eye and diseases of women.[193] Ebbell (1932) followed this up by mentioning that "the Ebers papyrus gives an extract of the whole of Egyptian medicine" because of its organized plan containing comprehensive medical matters (quoted in Leake 1940: 314). Ghalioungui (1973: 31) introduces Grapow's assertion of the comprehensive nature of the Ebers papyrus:

> Grapow (II, 104c) who studied these concordances in great detail remarked that, apart from two cosmetic preparations that appear in 3 papyri, none is common to more than two, and every repeated prescription exists in the Ebers papyrus, whereas no parallelism can be found between the Hearst and the Berlin, or between it and the London texts. This stressed the greater comprehensiveness of the Ebers papyrus that contains 4 or 5 times as much material as any of the others. Moreover, the close relationship between the Ebers and the Hearst papyri is shown by the fact that of the 105 duplicated texts, that are all found in the Ebers papyrus, 86 exist in the Hearst papyrus.

Nonetheless, Grapow (1955) also noticed an interesting fact in a comparison of orthography that though "the scribes of the Ebers and Hearst papyri simply followed the heterogeneous originals ... two papyri are not dependent on each other" (quoted in Leake 1940: 316).

Thus, for a statistical analysis, the Ebers papyrus may represent an ideal body of data because of its large volume and comprehensiveness. It seems preferable to use only the Eber papyrus, without including the other papyri in the analysis, on account of the number of duplications among the papyri that may lead to undesirable sampling bias (see p. 55). It would theoretically also be possible to apply an analysis to each medical papyrus separately, but the small volume of the other medical papyri (e.g. the Hearst papyrus comprises only 260 paragraphs, the Berlin papyrus contains 204 paragraphs and the London papyrus includes 61 paragraphs)[194] makes them appear to be unsuitable for a statistical analysis. Concerning the duplication of prescriptions contained in the Ebers papyrus itself (see p. 55), it is difficult to decide whether we should

the existence of a science that still escapes us."

[192] Ebers' opinion quoted in Dawson (1932–33: 34); Dawson (1932–33: 34) disagrees with this view of Ebers: "the Ebers papyrus is a miscellaneous collection of extracts and jottings collected from at least forty different sources. To call it, as Ebers did in his publication, a Hermetic Book, is entirely to mistake its nature and purpose."

[193] This classification of the clinical matter is reminiscent of the section "beginning of a compilation on the eyes" in the Ebers papyrus (Eb.336–431), and the Edwin Smith papyrus which comprises surgical treatments and the Kahun papyrus which treats diseases of women; See p. 23-4.

[194] These figures for paragraphs include incantation treatments, and the actual numbers of the paragraphs dealing with remedies in these papyri are less than these figures. The London papyrus, for example, includes only 25 medical paragraphs, and the rest is magical (Nunn 1996: 39); Westendorf (1999: 529–32) provides the summary of the proportion of the magical treatment attributed to each medical papyrus. According to it, the London papyrus has 66.7%; the Ramesseum papyrus IV with 73.3% includes many magical treatments while the Ebers papyrus with 1.7%, the Hearst papyrus with 3.5%) and the Berlin papyrus with 1.5% comprise much less magical treatment. The summery of the number and proportion of the prescription, instruction, prognosis and incantation text for each papyrus is also provided (Westendorf 1999: 95), and it reveals that the Ebers papyrus contains more than 800 prescriptions.

remove one of the duplicated prescriptions or just include all the prescriptions. I think it is better to include all prescriptions in the Ebers since sometimes we can find the same prescription repeated in a section on a different ailment, and it is difficult to judge if that is the result of simple error by the scribe or whether the same prescription was also efficient for another ailments.[195]

[195] For a discussion concerning the database construction and structure, see p. 73.

CHAPTER 6

Poly-pharmacological Perspective as a Device for Interpretation

6.1 Applying poly-pharmacological principles

Our second premise for the consideration of the efficacy of a statistical analysis of the Ebers papyrus is the validity of applying the poly-pharmacological principle to describe and understand the "environment" of the Egyptian prescriptions. The difficulties and problems in understanding Egyptian prescriptions from the "empirico-rational" and the "magico-religious" perspectives is mainly due to the integrity of science and religion in antiquity (see p. 21-2, 49-52). Another significant problem with applying the empirico-rational and magico-religious perspectives is that although they can point to the active principle of one or two materials in a prescription, they tend to ignore that of the effect other materials, even though Egyptian prescriptions can on average contain four or five materials. Also, the simple recognition of the empirico-rational and magico-religious element of the specific materials cannot describe the relationship with other materials included the prescription. This has often led to comments that most of the materials included in the prescriptions appear to be meaningless and worthless (see p. 5). Nevertheless, it seems that despite these short-comings of the two perspectives, we do not possess an effective alternative perspective that can lead to interpretations revealing the pharmacological principles behind Egyptian prescriptions. In the following, perspectives of poly-pharmacology in these two dimensions are discussed.

6.2 Poly-pharmacological perspectives of chemotherapy

Chemical active principle

Most modern drugs are produced based on knowledge of the pharmacological properties of chemicals, including purified chemicals from both plant extracts and synthetically produced ones. In medicines for common cold, for example, because no drug is yet known which can inhibit the virus that causes a cold, two or more drugs are put together to counteract and reduce the symptoms of a cold, but not its cause. An antihistamine is added to alleviate sneezing, runny nose and other allergic manifestations. Antihistamines produce a sleepy feeling as a depressant side effect, so caffeine is added to make the patient alert. A vasoconstrictor is added to contract blood vessels and thereby make room for the expansion of nasal airways so that the patient can breathe freely (Burger 1995: 40). Thus, the significance of pharmacology resides in its selection of biologically active chemical components in order to produce cooperative advantage from the combinations of them. As in this example, it is common to add chemicals that reduce undesirable side effects or counteract the near-toxic side effect of the main drug.

Nevertheless, the study of drugs from natural substances is fairly complex because one medicinal material can contain a number of active components. In the research of botanical medicine, an earlier method called "screening," which is still commonly employed to identify chemicals contained in a single plant, subject some major active components to a clinical test in which their prime property and efficacy are examined. White willow (*Salix alba*), for example, has been used from antiquity throughout the world as an antipyretic, analgesic and anti-inflammatory. The active chemical constituent of willow is salicin (glucoside of salicylic alcohol), identified in 1829, and salicin became a widely used medicine to treat fever, joint pain, rheumatism and so on. The analogous chemical compound acetylsalicylic acid was first chemically synthesised in 1853 and was soon mass-produced under the commercial name "Aspirin" (Silver *et al.* 1999: 2). Thus, willow extract is often regarded as the natural form of salicylic acid.[196] Willow was used in treatment for the "elimination

[196] Silver *et al.* (1999: 2) notes that in Germany, willow bark is often taken along with aspirin to enhance the therapeutic effects while minimizing side effects.

of swelling" (Eb.582) by the Egyptians. Acacia (*Acacia nilotica*) is characterized by its high concentration of tannin (phenolic compound). Tannin exhibits a property which dries mucus secretion and is commonly used internally for gastrointestinal disorders like diarrhoea and digestive tract inflammations. It also has an astringent and anti-microbial property and is also used externally to stop bleeding.[197] Acacia occurs not infrequently in Egyptian prescriptions for various ailments.

In this way, in research centres, many plants have been screened, and their chemicals have been identified, isolated and tested. Quite often the standardisation of a plant's pharmacological property has been made based on one or a few active marker ingredients of that plant, and often such information is given in the form of a list where the plant names and their marker chemical components are listed, often together with notes on their pharmacological benefits. This standardisation is methodologically practical and effective and also, to a certain degree, convincing. However, it is often criticised as a reductionist attitude since it ignores the important actions of other chemical components contained in the plant and the effects from the interaction between these chemical components. Chevallier (1996: 11) provides a simple example for the interaction of two ingredients in tea and coffee. According to him, tea and coffee contain approximately the same levels of caffeine. Tea, however, contains a much greater quantity of tannins, and these constituents reduce the amount of nutrients and drugs that are absorbed from the intestines into the blood-stream, and consequently less caffeine is absorbed. As a result, and true to most people's experience, tea is less stimulating than coffee. Also, Silver *et al.* (1999: 1) note that the high concentration of tannins in willow bark (8–20%) usually leads to gastrointestinal toxicity before therapeutic concentrations of salicylates are achieved.

There are numerous experience-based claims by the practitioners of botanical medicine claiming that the therapeutic effect of whole-plant extracts is in many cases superior to isolated compounds from the same plant. This phenomenon is commonly attributed to the synergetic effect resulting from the interactions of chemical components in the plant.[198] However, we do not have sufficient scientific knowledge to understand these complex biochemical interactions. We know several chemical constituents of aloe—which also has a long tradition of medicinal use and is commonly used orally for constipation and topically for external wounds and burns, including polysaccharides, lectins, anthracoid, salicylates, cholesterol, triglycerides, magnesium lactate and carboxypeptidase (Ang-Lee 2002: 7–8)—but we cannot understand and describe as a whole how these chemicals produce their pharmacological effects.[199]

Often the pharmaceutical chemicals of a plant need to be analysed according to separate parts of the plant because the active ingredients are not present in equal amounts in each part. The tannin of acacia, for instance, is typically highly concentrated in deseeded pods (50%), less in leaves (35%) and least in the inner bark (12–23%). Major parts of the plant that are commonly regarded as separate materials in botanical medicine include root, bulb, rhizome, tuber, bark, stem, leaf, flower, fruit, seed, gum and exudate. In many ancient Egyptian prescriptions, it is noticeable that the specific parts of a plant (as well as those of an animal) are indicated.

Dosage and effect

The dosage-response phenomenon is also an important concept of pharmacology, and it is usually recognised as being equally important as the selection of medicinal material because the dosage can directly influence the efficacy of the remedy.[200] Chevallier (2000: 11) provides us with an example showing the importance of the dosage for Chinese rhubarb (*Rheum palmatum*), which is a commonly used laxative containing anthraquinones that irritate the gut wall and stimulate bowel movement. This laxative effect, however, occurs only when large quantities of the herb are used. At lower doses other constituents, notably tannins, which dry and tighten up mucous membranes in the gut, have greater effect. As a result, Chinese rhubarb works in two apparently opposite ways depending on the dosage: as a laxative at moderate to high doses; and as a treatment for diarrhoea at a lower dose. Similarly, Bryant *et al.* (2003: 60) note that the intake of ginseng at low doses reduces blood pressure while higher doses can raise blood pressure. In Egyptian prescriptions we find the specification of dosages for materials in many cases. The significance of dosage in the prescriptions is indicated by the specification of the dosage always being written in red ink and also by the incantation in the Hearst papyrus titled as a spell for "the measuring cup on taking it in order to measure a prescription" (He.212). It states "As for this measuring utensil, I am measuring this prescription therewith. It is the measuring utensil which Horus measured his eye (remedy). It (the eye) was tested and I found (it) living, well and healthy. This prescription is measured with this measuring utensil in order to bring down therewith every sickness which is in his body ..." In Egyptian prescriptions, in most cases, the dosages are indicated by one stroke which represents one, and infrequently by two or more strokes. In

[197] Tannins are a very common ingredient in plants. Tannins are also known for their low toxic property at high dosage.

[198] Williamson (2000: 44) mentions that synergy broadly means "working together," and antagonism "working against each other."

[199] Ebadi (2002: 163) notes, for example, the significance of having a clear distinction between aloe latex and aloe gel because although "the leaves of the genus aloe are the source of two products", "they are quite different in their chemical composition and therapeutic properties" and in fact "These two products are obtained from two different specialized cells, latex from pericyclic cells and gel from parenchymatus cells."

[200] Two important concepts of dosage in present medicine are efficacy and potency. Efficacy refers to the magnitude of maximal response that can be produced from a drug (e.g. we can say drug A is more efficacious because it produces a higher maximal response), and potency refers to the amount of drug required to produce an effect (e.g. the more potent the drug, the lower the dose required for a given effect) (Adams *et al.* 2005: 59).

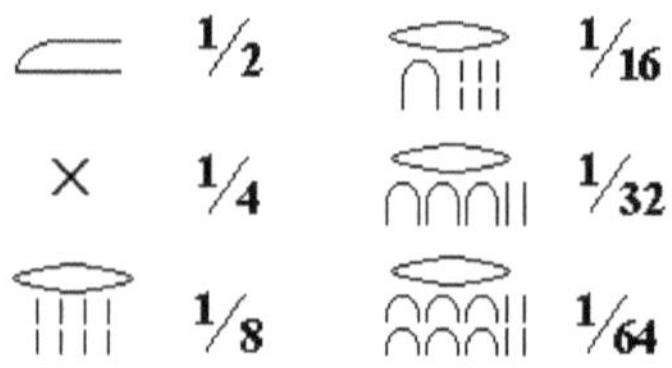

FIG. 9: FRACTIONAL NOTATIONS IN HIEROGLYPHICS

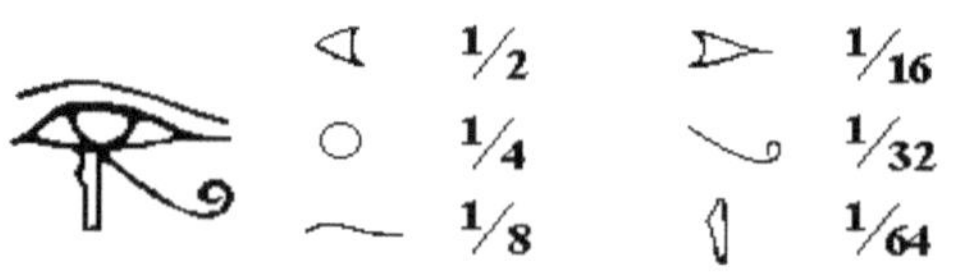

FIG. 10: FRACTIONAL NOTATIONS REPRESENTED WITH WDAT-EYE.

many cases, the minute quantities are indicated with two systems of fractional notation; the numeric expression of fractions and the symbolic notation of fractions with the *wḏ3t*-eye or "Eye of Horus" (Figs. 9 and 10).[201]

The indication of a stroke is often assumed to mean a piece of material or a relative proportion in a prescription, but it is also assumed to indicate a numeric expression of multiples of a certain amount of a unit. It is fractional notations that are generally understood as representing fractions of a certain quantity unit. The two systems are generally considered to represent the application of different units. In some cases, the unit of measurement is clearly noted in the prescription, as in those that use the unit *ḫnw* (e.g. Eb. 37, 42, 309, 323 and, in a different spelling, Eb.166, 281), but in most cases the unit is simply omitted. This omission makes the unit to be applied difficult to establish. Commonly suggested Egyptian units to be applied are *ḥḳt*, *ḫnw*, *ḏ*ᶜ and *r*, but the application of the unit has been interpreted in widely different ways by scholars. In addition, combinations of these dosage indications that are occasionally found in the prescriptions lead to different interpretations of the way quantities were calculated, and this results in considerable differences for the actual amount of the dosage specified in the prescription.[202] In a few cases, the quantity of the material is vaguely indicated by words like *šrj* or *nhy* ("little") (Eb.38, 212, 251) and *ᶜ3* ("much") (Eb.192 = 195).

There is no practical way for us to know the criteria for determining dosages in ancient Egypt, but Leake (1952: 41) notices that accurate measurements of materials occur particularly with costly materials such as frankincense or with substances that might be poisonous like toxic minerals, and he also notes that the remedies for internal administration are more carefully quantified. Leake (1952: 29–30) also comments that the Egyptian physicians might have recognised that drugs given by mouth have a more general systematic effect, and the intensity of the drug action in general varies directly with the quantity of the drug given.[203] In relation to this, Germer (1993: 78) provides a comment on wine: "Wine was often taken as a base for the prescription but the amount of wine was so small that the patient could not have become drunk."

Prospects for future research

As discussed above, an understanding of a prescription consisting of natural substances requires consideration of numerous complex factors including the chemicals and their pharmaceutical properties, interactions among chemicals, the ratio of concentration of the chemical in

[201] In Egyptian myth the eye of Horus was gouged into fragments by his wicked rival Seth, and his eye was restored by remedy and magic. Being associated with this notion, each part of the eye of Horus represents a fraction and their total makes nearly one. For fractures, see of the Eye of Horus, see Gardiner (1957: 197); The pharmacological symbol ℞ used today is sometimes assumed to be a schematic derivation from the Eye of Horus (Weeks 1995: 1796).

[202] The metrology of the medical papyri was treated as early as 1875 by Ebers (1875: 18), and Griffith (1891) provided a foundational work for a study on this subject. A Number of different interpretations have been made, and totally different values for Egyptian pharmacological metrology have been suggested. One interpretation is based on the conversion table of the Rhind mathematical papyrus which dates from the same period with many of the preserved medical papyri (18th Dynasty) that provides some indication of the probable amount of the units. It seems generally accepted that *ḫnw* amounts to around 450 to 480 ml and *r*, being 1/32 of *ḫnw*, to around 14 to 15 ml (Leake 1952: 19–20; Sigerist 1951: 337; Manniche 1989: 63; Nunn 1996: 141–2); Westendorf (1999: 521–4) applies the unit *ḥk3t* and *r* for the interpretation of the Egyptian medical dosage. He notes that *ḥk3t* is equal to 4800 ccm and *r* is equal to 15 ccm, and the dosages based on *r* (1/2 *r* = 7.5 ccm, 1/4 *r* = 3.75 … 1/128 *r* = 0.117 ccm) "entspricht dem Satz von 7 Meßbechern (dbH-Gefäßen ?) aus der 18.Dynastie mit einem jeweil halbierten Fassungsvermögen von 6 bis 0,1 ccm" (Westendorf 1999: 523). Nunn (1996: 141) provides a picture showing the small volume measures from the Petrie Museum (UC 26315); Estes (1993: 96) comments that *wḏ3t* notations are probably mean simply as proportional parts of the final whole. Nevertheless, continuing disagreement with this interpretation is noticeable. Pommerening (2003) recently proposed an alternative interpretation from a pharmacologist's perspective. She first describes and summarises the quite different interpretation of medical metrology of Ebbell (1937), the *Grundriß*, Bardinet (1995) and Westendorf (1999) (Pommerening 2003: 3–7). She notes "Die frühere Korrelation im *Grundriß* hätte zu einer Tagesration von nur 100 ml geführt—einer allzu geringen Menge, wenn man eine pharmakologische Wirkung erzielen möchte. Die Auflösung der Bruchquanten in definierte Volumenanteile macht es nun erstmal möglich, die pharmakologischen Wirksamkeiten der altägyptischen Arzneimittel aus heutiger Sicht zu beurteilen" (Pommerening 2003: 12). The new interpretation by Pommerening (2003) is that the capacity markings of the two complete vessels, with marked volumes of 1 and 1/2 *ḫnw* and 1, 1/2 , 1/4 , 1/8 , 1/16 , 1/32 and 1/64 *ḏ*ᶜ, allow all relevant volumes to be measured which are required in the preparations mentioned in extant medical papyri.

[203] Leake (1952: 29) notes that in the Ebers papyrus, 86% of internal administrations is quantified and 62% for external application. The tendency to give the dosage indication, particularly in the internal administrations can be confirmed from the observation that 81% of internal remedies are quantified while this applies to only 35% of external applications in the Hearst papyrus, and in the Berlin Papyrus 68% of oral remedies are quantified while this is the case for only 12% of topical applications.

a particular part of the substance and dosages applied. In the current stage of our science, however, we cannot fully understand and illustrate the precise mechanism of pharmaceutical actions, even of a single natural substance. Therefore, assessing the actual pharmaceutical effect of a remedy produced from several natural substances remains unrealistic at the present time. Nevertheless, Wagner (2000: 35) maintains a positive attitude toward the investigation of the complex botanical medicine:

> In order to investigate complex systems such as plant drugs and phytopreparations, which consist of many bioactive compounds, the suggestion of the philosopher Descartes should be followed. He proposed that complex systems that cannot easily be analysed by simple means might be investigated by examining the individual parts of the system. In this way, it is hoped that a rational explanation for a whole will emerge. In other words, more-or-less reductionistic research must be carried out with an awareness, however, that this strategy will never quite explain the entire efficacy of the complete complex of active compounds. The term 'the whole is more than the sum of all its individual parts' is certainly applicable to phytopharmaceuticals.

Research in botanical pharmacology has been advancing at an ever-accelerating rate, and many reports and articles are published every year in medical journals and the more recent computerised articles, and the accessibility to such publications via the internet provides us with greater opportunity to consult recent studies.[204] A notable recent innovative investigation method is computational drug analysis in which the predicting of "drug-likeness" are made by a computer.[205] Just as reappraisals of Egyptian prescriptions have occurred each time a pharmaceutically active compound of a material was identified and found to have been used by the Egyptians, current investigations also provide us with useful information for understanding and interpreting Egyptian pharmacology.[206]

Synergistic effect of poly-pharmacological medicine

On the whole, we need always to be aware that one material can produce several different effects and can be used in different treatments, as in the case of honey whose antimicrobial property is regularly used for wounds and burns but can also be rationally used for contraception because of its effect of diminishing the motility of spermatozoa (Kh.22) (Bardis 1967: 1). The same is true of a single substance which contains many active components such as acacia whose tannins are commonly regarded as its active component, but the lactic acid anhydride from the gum of the acacia has a spermicidal capacity (Eb.783) (Bardis 1968: 2; Cole 1986: 30). Banov (1965: 1041) compares the Egyptian use of honey for an anorectal disease (Cht.9) with the application of sugar to promote the reduction of the prolapsed bowel of procidentia through the osmotic removal of water today. Thus we can identify many pharmacological properties for a material.

In addition, we have to be aware of the unexplained overall efficacy of a remedy from natural substances. The poly-pharmacological effect produced from a selected combination of materials is not always additive, but different ingredients can be taken for different functions, and these functions by the sub-active principle may result in greater efficacy, the synergistic effect. Another important concept in the poly-pharmacological principle is a function of the material called the "adaptogenic" effect. The adaptogenic effect is attributed to materials which can reduce undesirable side-effects produced by the chief or other material, often through demonstrating opposing action to them, and they contribute to the body's ability to respond to stresses (Bryant 2003: 60).

6.3 Poly-pharmacological perspective of systematic theory of medicine

There may be objections to discussing the pharmacological theory of Egyptian medicine in a context of systematic theory, which is usually considered to be present only in advanced medicine. But the pharmacological concept of systematic medicine can actually provide us with some meaningful poly-pharmacological perspectives when considering the Egyptian prescriptions. The essence of treatment in systematic theory is to cure the disease, which is the result of excess or deficiency of bodily constitutions, by restoring the lost harmonious balance on the bases of the allopathic principle in which a remedy with the opposite property is given against the disease (see p. 17). Although this fundamental concept may appear quite

[204] There are several useful electronic databases of articles of medicine such as MEDILINE, PubMed and EMBASE. A search can be undertaken using the names of individual plants and primary terms for search like "antibacterial" or "antiinflammatory."

[205] One problem of the strategy of isolating and testing botanical chemicals is its inefficiency of time. It can often take 6 months to isolate and structurally analyse a chemical from a plant, and this approach requires a prohibitively long time equivalent to a lifetime for a researcher. With reference to its efficacy, Clark *et al.* (2000: 49) states "Much has been written recently concerning the impact of combinatorial chemistry and high-throughput screening (HTS) on drug discovery. However, there is growing realization that, given the vase size of organic chemical space (possibly $>10^{18}$ compounds), drug discovery cannot be reduced to a simple 'synthesize-and-test' lottery ... there is currently much interest in the development and application of computational methods for predicting 'drug-likeness.' Such methods could be applied to *virtual* compounds or libraries permitting the rapid and cost effective elimination ..."

[206] Recent research on botanical medicine provides precise and specific analyses, but ironically often this leads to difficulties in applying the information to an understanding of Egyptian prescriptions mainly due to the different concept of disease in modern and ancient medicine. We can safely apply the chemical properties like "antiparasitic" or "antimicrobial," but it would be difficult for a property like "immuno-stimulating" or "anti-cancer"; we also need to consider that since the Egyptian prescriptions typically have instructions to be applied for four days, it may be better that we apply the confirmation of efficacy which emerges in a relatively short period of time when we assume the rationality of the Egyptian prescription based on it.

simple, its actual pharmacological manipulation requires complex considerations of the precise nature of each disease and individual substance. In principle, in Greek, Chinese or Āyurvedic medicine, nothing is regarded as purely hot or cold, or as having a specific quality of any kind, but all things are regarded as consisting of a mixture of several properties in varying concentrations.[207] An ingredient can, for example, have the primary property of coolness with also some heating property, and then another counteractive ingredient can be employed to nullify the undesired property of heating with the property of the other ingredient. This pharmacological principle is known as the "contra-indicated ingredient" (or "antagonizing effect"), and it is with this principle that the poly-pharmacological remedies are prescribed so that the whole property of the remedy is properly adjusted so as to be suitable as a treatment.

1	**limit**	**unlimited**
2	**odd**	**even**
3	**one**	**plurality**
4	**right**	**left**
5	**male**	**female**
6	**resting**	**moving**
7	**straight**	**crooked**
8	**light**	**darkness**
9	**good**	**bad**
10	**square**	**oblong**

TABLE 6: "TABLE OF TEN OPPOSITES" WHICH ARISTOTLE SETS APART FROM THE REST OF THE PYTHAGOREAN NUMBER THEORY (BASED ON BURKERT 1972: 51).

Cosmology and medicine

The dualistic cosmic theory provides us with a clearer understanding of the essential idea of neutralizing by opposing qualities. The foundation of the dualistic cosmology in ancient Greece can be traced back to the numerology of Pythagoras (580–489 BC). In the Pythagorean doctrine, mathematics is regularly emphasised as the primary principle of cosmology. In it, the alternation of "even" and "odd" in the number series is assigned to correspond to the antithesis, "limit" and "unlimited," and the resulting theory is that the number is harmony as that which transcends the opposition of "limit" and "unlimited." This concept of numerology was used in the attempts to illustrate the nature of universe. Its significance was asserted in a passage of Iamblichus (*Iam. Comm. Math.* sc.25 p. 78, 8–21), which is obviously derived from Aristotle's book on the Pythagoreans, that "whoever wishes to comprehend the true nature of actual things, should turn his attention to these things, the numbers and proportions, because it is by them that everything is made clear" (Burkert 1972: 50). The dualistic cosmology was formulated primarily on the basis of this numerological concept, and it was expanded by including all aspects of nature within its dualistic cosmic model through a command of analogy and recognition of antithesis (Table 6).[208]

The Greeks' understanding and description of harmony in the universe based on numerology is also expressed in their idea of cosmic music. Their musicology is formed on a basis of musical intervals, rhythms and velocities determined by numeral ratio and proportion, and it assumes the "harmony of the spheres" through a musical harmony based on the coherence and harmony of numbers. Therefore, just as the opposing qualities of numbers could produce a harmonious cosmological sphere, so the harmonious state of the universe was regarded as comprising constitutions of antithetical properties. The intrinsic part of the Pythagorean doctrine is characterised by its recognition of opposite extremes that are created through the extraction of the middle. This doctrine, however, leads to wide-ranging discussions among the Greek philosophers in antiquity, and it is frequently the subject of criticism which points to its occasional unreasonable categorising of things into opposing groups and its failure to recognise the significant existence of a median position.[209] Through the discussions in the Pythagorean tradition, Philolaus mentions that "existing things must be, all of them, either limiting, or unlimited, or both limiting and unlimited; but they would not be unlimited only (or limiting only?). Since, however, they are clearly neither made of limiting (constituents) only or of unlimited only, it is therefore obvious that from both limiting and unlimited (constituents) the cosmos

[207] Hippocratic text (*On Ancient Medicine* XV) states "I do not think they have ever discovered anything that is purely 'hot' or 'cold', 'dry' or 'wet', without it sharing some other qualities" (Chadwick 1978: 79); The complex multiplicity of medicinal properties of a botanical material is referred to, for instance, in a Hippocratic text which reads "The qualities of vegetables are as follows. Garlic warms, passes well by stool and by urine, and is good for the body though bad for the eyes. For making a considerable purgation of the body it dulls the sight … The radish moistens through melting the phlegm by its sharpness, but the leaves do so less. The root is bad for arthritis, and it repeats and is hard to digest … Coriander is hot and astringent; it stops heartburn, and when eaten last also causes sleep. Lettuce is rather cooling before it has its juice, but sometimes it produces weakness in the body. Anise is hot and astringent, and the smell of it stops sneezing … Mint warms, passes easily by urine, and stops vomiting; if eaten often it melts the seed and makes it run, preventing erections and weakening the body" etc (*On Regimen* II, 54) (trans. Jones 1931: 329–31).

[208] Aristotle (*Metaphysics*, 986a 13–21) mentions about the Pythagorean doctrine "Now they too clearly consider number to be a first principle, both as material substrate for existing things and as modifications and states of these things they consider that the elements (*stoicheia*) of number are the Odd and the Even, the former being limited and the latter unlimited. The One (unity) proceeds from both (it being both odd and even), number proceeds from unity and, as we mentioned the whole universe is number" (Philip 1966: 47).

[209] For instance, Aristotle (*Metaphysics*, 1091a 12–18) mentions "It is absurd and indeed impossible to erect a theory ascribing coming-to-be (*genesis*) to eternal things. Yet without a doubt the Pythagorians do so. They say that when the One has come into existence, by being put together from plane surfaces or surface limits (*chrois*) or seeds or some unspecified constituent, at once Limit draws in to itself and limits the nearest parts of the Unlimited" (Philip 1966: 50).

and the things in it were harmoniously put together ..." (Burkert 1972: 251).

There are considerable similarities between the Greek dualistic cosmology and the Chinese *yin-yang* theory. Certainly, the *yin-yang* theory emphasises medium qualities between *yin* and *yang*. It describes, for example, *yin* as possessing a *yin*-in-*yin* phase (mature *yin*), but there can also be yang contained in *yin*, and in a similar way, there is *yang*-in-*yang* and *yin*-in-*yang*. The advanced forms of cosmology have come about through an expansion from dualism to pluralism in the recognition of primary cosmic constituents. Greek cosmology has four symbolic cosmic constituents, and there are five in Chinese cosmology. The notable feature in the formation of both these cosmologies is the structure of the systematised mechanical relationship among the constituents that form a geometric pattern of correspondence, in which an excess or deficiency of constituents can be neutralised, producing the equilibrium of the cosmos (see p. 16-7). Just as a dualistic cosmology can serve as a basis for the description and understanding of the whole of nature, a pluralistic cosmology, through its synchronic integrity of all natural phenomena, becomes the primary principle for the understanding of the universe.

There is an interesting parallel between Greek and Chinese cosmic music in that the Greek lyre has four strings which correspond to the four rhythms of seasons which in turn is related to the elements, and the five notes of Chinese music correspond to five seasons and phases (Burkert 1972: 356). Medicine is one of the components of this systematic cosmological theory, concerned with understanding the human body, disease and healing. Thus, medicine as part of a systematic theory necessarily emphasises the significance of the balance of bodily constitutions, and pharmacological treatment is based on the application of a remedy that can counterbalance an excess or deficiency in these bodily constituents.

Notion of socio-politics and medicine

In pharmacology of systematic medicine, each individual medicinal material is assumed to have a primary property which is its cosmic constituent, and it is also assigned some other properties of a lesser degree. Usually, in drug designing, a chief material which is necessary to counteract the lack of harmony among the bodily constituents is chosen first, and then secondary material is employed which aims to enhance and support the property of the chief material or to reduce or eliminate the undesirable qualities of the chief material. This method of design operates quite systematically through the calculations of the properties, of enhancing and neutralising materials, so that the quality of a remedy as a whole is suitably adjusted. More often, further complex designing is undertaken by combining several materials for a remedy.[210] In one tradition of Chinese pharmacology, this principle of drug design is commonly illustrated by the additionally associating socio-political concepts. By this, a primary therapeutic material is defined as "sovereign (or ruler)" and several secondary materials are assigned as "ministers," and materials which play only supporting roles are called "assistants" followed by materials called "aids" (Unschuld 1985: 115).[211] And when the prescriptions for the remedies are written down, the "sovereign" material is written first followed by the "minister" down to the "aid," and this sequence in the listing of materials enables other medical practitioners to understand the function played by each material in the remedy. Weeks (1976–78: 297) notices a comparable feature in the Egyptian records of prescriptions in that there is a tendency in most prescriptions of the Ebers papyrus to arrange the materials in a hierarchical order: the principal ingredients are listed toward the beginning of a prescription, less important ingredients follow, and any liquid medium used to facilitate ingestion or application is given last (see p. 78-9).[212] Actually, even with a quick scan of Egyptian prescriptions, we can observe that the material that serves as the vehicle of the remedy, such as a liquid or semi-liquid substance, tends to appear in the last part or at the end of the material list.

Forming an association between medicine and socio-political principles is also a noticeable feature in Greek and Chinese medicine. Alcmaeon of Croton in the fifth century BC describes health as being maintained through balance as a "democracy" and disease was a "monarchy" in which an excess of one quality overwhelmed the other, and he uses the word *isonomia* for "balance," the same is used for equality in political rights (King 2001: 8). The connection between socio-politics and medicine in China is showed in a passage from the "Basic Question" of the *Inner Canon*: "The cardiac system is the office of the monarch; consciousness issues from it. The pulmonary system is the office of the minister-mentors; oversight and supervision issue from it. The hepatic system is the office

[210] Guili (1997: 13–14) introduces seven conditions under which practitioners of Chinese medicine select drugs: (1) treating an illness with one drug alone; (2) two kinds of drugs with similar properties used in combination to reinforce each other's action; (3) two or more ingredients used in combination, one being the principal substance while the rest play a subsidiary role to reinforce the action of the former; (4) mutual restraining effect of different ingredients to weaken or neutralize each other's toxicity or side-effect; (5) the property of one ingredient to neutralize the toxicity of another ingredient; (6) the property of one ingredient to weaken the action of another ingredient; (7) incompatibility that severe side-effect may result when two incompatible ingredients are used in combination. Guili (1997: 14) summarises that combination of drugs may "interpromote" the curative effect or may "interrestrain" to decrease each other's toxicity or side-effect.

[211] For a concept of structure of forming formula in Chinese medicine, see Qingye (1998: 12).

[212] Weeks (1976–78: 297) mentions this fact may be a useful clue in identifying unknown material names that "For example, Grapow's group 4, which contains prescriptions 188–207, is devoted to the treatment of gastro-intestinal disorders. Where the drug names and something of their physiological effect is known to us, the primary goal of each of these prescriptions was to facilitate the evacuation of the stomach and bowels by means of powerful emetics or purgatives. In most cases, the emetic or purgative agent is the first or second drug given in prescription. It seems likely, therefore, that if, of the drugs listed in first or second position in any group 4 prescription, some of them are not yet translated, we still can assume that one of them is probably an emetic or purgative."

of the General; planing issues from it. The gall bladder system is the office of the rectifiers; decision issue from it … (and so on for twelve systems of body functions associated with internal organs). It will not do for these twelve offices to lose their coordination" (Sivin 1995: 7).

Egyptian cosmology and systematic theory

When we study a cosmology based on a systematic theory, we notice certain similarities with the Egyptian cosmology and its notion of *mꜣ*ʿ*t* (see p. 50-2). There can be three prime dynamics that contribute to forming a cosmology in a systematic theory: analogy, antithesis and the law of the universe that maintains the order and harmony of the cosmos. Possible cases of the Egyptian use of analogy have already been discussed in the examples of Egyptian homeopathic treatment (see p. 37-8). Concerning the recognition of antithesis, the notion of duality in nature—such as "day" and "night", "light" and "dark", "living" and "dead", "male" and "female", "right" and "left", "hot" and "cold", "good" and "bad", and "justice" and "evil"—is identical to what is commonly held in most cultures.[213] Such recognition of antithesis is also evident in the Egyptian medical texts in such cases as "The breath of life enters into the right ear and the breath of death enters into the left ear" (Eb.854f; Eb.856g)[214] and in the method of how to recognise milk that is bad (Eb.788) and that is good (Eb.796). The significant similarity is the emphasis on the harmony of the universe found in both the cosmic equilibrium of a systematic theory and the Egyptian notion of the cosmic order *mꜣ*ʿ*t*. The application of this same principle to the understanding of all phenomena through the principle of macrocosm and microcosm can also be observable. The divine force was not arbitrary but the force to keep *mꜣ*ʿ*t* in all phases of heavenly and earthly systems. From this comparison, disclosing essential similarities in the recognition of cosmology, one may argue Egyptians were very near to establishing the formation of systematic theory. However, it is also to be noticed that there is a lack of concrete evidence to assume the existence of systematic theory in ancient Egypt because their writings always keep silence in their intrinsic knowledge of fact. The circumspection and restoration of lost theory base on conjecture inducted by comparison with other culture's theory is dangerous and can be erroneous, and thus it is particularly difficult to draw broad conclusions on this matter, and it is certain that "argumentum a silentio" is risky (Ghalioungui 1968: 100–1) (see p. 71 n. 216).

The crucial point here is that we do not know if the Egyptians were able to combine the analogous and antithetical elements into a systematised structure of correspondences where elements can interact and neutralise each other, producing the mutually balanced state that constitutes the harmony of the universe. Also, there are essential differences between the cosmology of a systematic theory and the Egyptian cosmology in that the cosmology of the former is based on the deductive science of natural components represented by abstract symbols whereas the latter cosmology consists of forces of divinities.

Scholars often note the significance of contributions from the scientific tradition of the neighbouring, older civilisations of Egypt and of Babylonia, in the areas of mathematics, geometry and astronomy, that are also regarded as essential components needed in the Greeks' achievement of elaborating and formulating a systematic theory. Saunders (1963: 2) states "in the case of science and medicine we must ask ourselves the question: what preceded the scientific revolution which began in Greece during the sixth century B.C." As already mentioned (see p. 68), although Hippocrates is generally held to be the representative who led to the invention of the theory of four humours in medicine, we can trace back its origin to the Pythagorean doctrine of the sixth century BC, where we find the primary pair of bodily powers—"hot" and "cold", and "dry" and "wet", "sweet" and "sour", etc. already included in the dualistic principle of its doctrine. Pythagoras himself is reported to have visited Egypt and studied there as a pupil of one Un-nefer of Heliopolis (Saunders 1963: 14). There are several more Greek scholars who we know studied in Egypt including Alcmaeon of Croton (*fl.* 530 BC), the younger contemporary of Pythagoras, who greatly reinforced the scientific side of medicine and is said to have derived his pneumanist doctrine from Egypt, and Thales of Miletos (*c.* 624–544 BC), who reputedly founded the Ionic school of medicine, and was a pupil of Egyptian priests, and Eudoxos of Cnidos (*c.* 408–355 BC) who also studied under the Egyptian Chinuphis (Saunders 1963: 14). This shows that Greeks were keen to learn from Egypt and that many early scholars visited Egypt. The fame of Egypt's learning remained even after the flourishing of Greek science, as we can see by Aristotle's (383–322 BC) visit to Egypt and Plato's visit to Heliopolis around 390 BC, and even the Roman physician Galen (129–?199 AD) studied in Alexandria and wrote in his work (*de Composit. Medicament*, v, 2) that Greek physicians still visit the library of the school of Memphis to consult medical works (Ghalioungui 1973: 66; Reymond 1984: 198). Can we then conclude that the early Greek scholars knew they learnt from Egypt? Can we deduce the extent of knowledge they acquired there and that it was applied to the formation and development of their own science? Although there are indicators that suggest that Greek physicians were influenced by Egyptian ideas, the paucity of evidence leaves room for discussion when it comes to the identification of the precise areas of Egyptian influence on Greek medicine.[215]

[213] Frankfort (1961: 73) notes Egyptians believed the universe to contain opposing forces in perennial equilibrium that "Evil, then, had its appointed place, counterbalanced—and kept in place—by good."

[214] This view of evil left side may be an early example for the notion of "sinister."

[215] As Saunders (1963: 3) notes "Indeed it is possible to find statements, without further specification or adequate documentation, that both the pneumatic and humoral doctrines of Greek medicine were derived from Egypt," certainly we can find interpretations of the Egyptian medicine based on the Greek style systematic theory, but in the current situation

There is room for more speculation. Apart from the historical or cultural links with Greece or the similarities between Egyptian and Greek medicine, cross-cultural medical study can tell us that there are no grounds for the idea that medicine is an independent entity, rather, medicine is an integral component of the whole set of cultural beliefs. But how are notions of analogy, antithesis, Egyptian cosmology with its concept of *mꜣꜥt* and the socio-political concept related to the elaboration of Egyptian medicine?[216] There must have certainly been significant dynamics associated with medical principles, just as in Greece, China and India, and we may speculate that these dynamics played some significant role in the formation of the principles of Egyptian medicine. There is, however, no way to know what these were like. We may sympathise with Ghalioungui (1961: 20) who laments:

> Their knowledge was certainly more extensive than we might imagine. Only if the ruined temples and 'house of life' could rise again, if the destroyed papyri could be restored, or if the scholars who restricted their teaching by the spoken word to the initiated could be resuscitated, could we form an exact idea of their achievement. But from what we know, we can say that it was a great step in the liberation of man, in fact, the first attempt in history of free science from magic.

So many Egyptian medical ideas must be lost. The medical writings must have been full of these ideas but it is impossible to re-establish them.[217]

6.4 Poly-pharmacological principle as a perspective

Through the considerations above, it has become clear that it would be difficult to effectively describe and understand the poly-pharmacological features and the patterns exhibited in Egyptian prescriptions based on the poly-pharmacological principle of both chemotherapeutic medicine and the systematic theory of medicine, mainly due to the complexity of chemical interactions and the medical anthropological difficulties in the comparison of medicines of different cultures.

The study of poly-pharmacological principles, however, has the potential to bring forth some important facts as to how the medicinal materials can be assigned different functions, and how they are at times not directly related to the treatment itself. Also, the notions of the "adaptogenic effect" and the "contra-indicated ingredient" alert us to the possibility that employing medicinal materials which can produce the opposite effect to that intended by the treatment is not at all irrational in poly-pharmacological prescriptions, for such ingredients help reduce the bodily stress from the drug or enhance the whole value of the remedy.

such an interpretation appears to be overenthusiastic and speculative (see p. 71 n. 217). Ghalioungui (1967a: 47) states "mais l'on ne peut nier l'originalité de l'apport grec qui a fécondé ces idées," but Ghalioungui (1984: 185) notes "It is difficult to tell how deeply these two scientists (Herophilus and Erasistratos) might have been inspired by stray copies of the Pharaonic 'Beginning of the Physician's Secret' or of other papyri kept in the libraries of Alexandria and Memphis for, according to Galen, Greek physicians still studied there in the second century AD. But some notions seem curiously common to Alexandrian and Pharaonic physicians: the relation of the heart to the pulse, the notion of pulse rate and its importance in diagnosis, and the concept of healthy and morbid circulating matter of different kinds. There is no doubt, however, that this remarkable renaissance of the Greek miracle in Alexandria was ignited by the impact of Greek logic on the mixture of mysticism and empiricism that characterised Egyptian thought ..." Ghalioungui (1968: 103–4) also comments "Yet, early works of the Corpus Hippocraticum still understood phlegm and bile in the Cnidian sense. The Hippocratic and Galenic theory of the four humours was a late construction, and elaboration of the early concept of circulating pathogens fused with the love and hate theory of Empedocles and with the Pythagorean concern with numbers. Health emerged from this crucible as a state of equilibrium between four contraries, and disease as a disturbance of that balance. The idea of equilibrium suited the followers of Empedocles' love and hate, and the number four was after the heart of the Pythagoreans, whose master probably heard from the Heliopolitan priest with whom he studied that the universe is composed of four hermetic elements, heaven, earth, water, and air." Ghalioungui (1967a: 48) also assumed the developmental formation of a medicine through the interaction of Egypt and Greek cultures in such a way that "... Elles ne témoignent pas moins d'un essai de reflexion raisonnée qui n'a pu s'aventurer bien loin, néanmoins, à cause de l'hésitation des Egyptiens devant la spéculation pure. Cette aversion peut avoir été la raison de l'arrêt de la médecine égyptienne après sa première floraison sous l'Ancien Empire. Aux antipodes de la pensée égyptienne, l'engouement grec pour les constructions rationnelles finit, après l'âge d'or d'Hippocrate, par transformer leur médecine en un pur exercice de dialectique dont ils avaient de la peine à se dégager. Dans le domaine de la médecine, la raison et l'expérience doivent aller de pair. Et ce n'est peut-être pas une coïncidence que la magnifique floraison de savants qui valut à Alexandrie de devenir l'école du monde ait eu lieu justement dans cette ville quand la sagesse égyptienne y rencontra la logique des Grecs." More recently, Stephan (2001: 267; 2005: 98) argues that the medical knowledge and practice of Greek physicians, notably "(1) Hippokrates und die Schule von Kos mit der Humoralpathologie, (2) Empedokles und die Schule von Agrigent mit der Viersäftelehre, (3) Euryphon und die Schule von Knidos mit der Lehre von den umherziehenden Krankheitsstoffen (perittoma) and (4) Herophilus und die Schule von Alexandria mit der Pulsmessung," were built upon Egyptian foundations.

216 Banu (1967: 126–8), after a discussion of the Egyptian concept of *mꜣꜥt*, states "Sans doute, un tel tableau permet à l'imagination d'associer de la façon la plus libre possible les notions de cosmique et d'humain." But his argument regarding the pulse examination that the Edwin Smith papyrus (Sm.1) explains with a term *ipt* ("count") (see p. 30) still appears speculative, when he states that "le cours ordonné de la nature intime du corps lui apparaît comme possédant un *rythme* (le pouls). Mais il pense aussi au fait qu'il y a de même une rythmicité cosmique: la succession rythmique des années, des saisons, le mouvement cyclique des astres"; Porter (1997: 49–50) states that in ancient Egypt, "illness was a matter of imbalance which could be restored to be equilibrium by supplication, spells and rituals. Thus, someone struck blind might invoke a god: 'Ptah, the lord of Truth, has turned his justice against me; he has rightly chastised me." This interpretation of Egyptian medicine along the same lines as the Greek medical principle is probably based on the similarity seen in the concept of the harmony of universe, in Egyptian *mꜣꜥt*, and Greek cosmology, but the lack of textual evidence in the Egyptian medical texts to support the presence of such a medical theory in Egypt invalidates this conclusion; Gordon and Schwabe (2004) also repeatedly assume the association of the concept of *mꜣꜥt* and Egyptian biomedical notion in their work.

217 Prioreschi (2003: 156) notes that "we must consider the possibility that the more limited breadth and depth of Egyptian naturalistic medicine could be due to the paucity of surviving documents ... A comparable situation would exist if all that had survived of Greek medicine were 377 lines (the length of Smith papyrus) of the Hippocratic Corpus, 2289 lines (the length of the Ebers papyrus) of Galen, and a few fragmentary texts dealing mainly with Aesculapian medicine. If this were the case, there is no doubt that Greek medicine would appear to us to be much less important."

PART 3

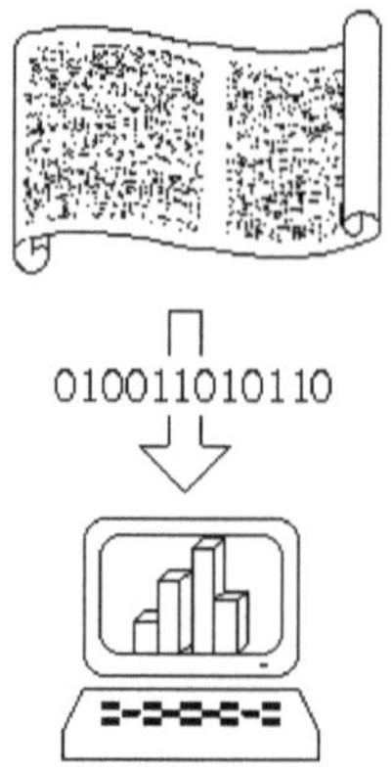

Demonstration

In this part of the study, the methodology of a statistical analysis of the Ebers papyrus is presented. The method of database construction and the statistical tests to be applied are introduced first, then several technical problems in accommodating the data from the Egyptian prescription into the database and some necessary premises for analysis of the extracted dataset are discussed. In a final step, selected results and commentaries are presented.

CHAPTER 7

A Statistical Analysis of the Ebers Papyrus

The fundamental question that comes to one's mind when studying Egyptian medicine is whether any meaningful information can be derived from examining the patterns of the materials found throughout prescriptions recorded in the Egyptian medical papyri. Some scholars point to the existence of specific patterns and tendencies in the formulation of remedies. Leake (1940: 320) notes in regard to Larkey's conclusion that "Dr. Larkey has made an exhaustive study of the different disease conditions in which the various drug materials are recommended. It is his opinion that there is consistency in the type of used recommended." The significance of this "consistency," however, can be questioned due to the fragmentary nature of the medical writings (see p. 5, 54-6). In Greek medical writings, the Hippocratic corpus can be regarded as a representative legacy of Greek medicine. Similarly, the Ebers papyrus can be regarded as representative of Egyptian medicine.[218] Unlike the Hippocratic corpus, which can be seen to reveal primary medical theories as well as a diversity of medical ideas, the Ebers papyrus does not allow us to access the underlying Egyptian medical ideas that guided the physicians' preparation of remedies. If we do assume that the consistencies found in the patterns of Egyptian prescription have significance, we would be more inclined to regard them as an unchangeable "core reality"—to borrow a term from statistics (see p. 6)—that is derived from the Egyptians' early establishment of medicine and preserved by their conservative traditionalism. The interpretation of "consistencies and patterns" in the pharmacological sense, however, is difficult because of the complexity of medicine consisting as it does of natural substances as well as of poly-pharmacological principles.

It is certain, however, that some detailed studies of a specific material and its pattern of occurrence in prescriptions could lead to some meaningful suggestions (see p. 3, 46 n. 121). In this respect, systematic statistical operations applied to the Ebers papyrus may reveal more specific consistencies and particular patterns, and we may obtain some useful data. Weeks (1976–78: 299) states "... we still have so much to learn of this practice that even something as simple as a sorting program will help us learn more about it."

7.1 Methodology for a statistical analysis

A variety of methodologies for a statistical approach to the Ebers papyrus are conceivable, but to promote full-scale analyses it is practical to accommodate the data-items from the papyrus into a database before commencing any statistical approach. For the purpose of the present study, employing the relational database model is appropriate because it can not only accommodate and structurally represent the relationships of different kinds of data-items but the applications of a relational database are also usually equipped with a special programming language called SQL (Structured Query Language), and this allows the investigator to set criteria from which specific datasets can be derived.[219] Also, the data manipulations a relational database can perform, may include some of the arithmetic calculations needed for the statistical analyses. The datasets derived through SQL are often transferred into a spread-sheet type database or other statistical applications like SPSS, Simstat and WordStat that provide specialised functions for statistical analyses. Several techniques relating to statistical tests can be included in the analysis such as frequency distribution and cross-tabulation which will yield distribution patterns. For testing and measuring the specific relationship of two or more elements, bivariate or multivariate data analysis including chi-square, ANOVA and a correlation test can be used.[220] A correspondence

[218] For the discussion of the issue of whether the Ebers papyrus is representative, see Chapter 5; The premise behind using only the Ebers papyrus for an analysis has already been discussed, see p. 62-3.

[219] Access, the relational database application provided by Microsoft, allows us to use VBA (Visual Basic for Application) which enables the user more flexible data manipulation.

[220] For a basic concept of bivariate and multivariate data analysis, see

analysis is useful for recognition of the comprehensive associations of several elements.

Technical difficulties and problems

Notable technical difficulties that occur in the process of accommodating prescription data into a database and also in operating statistical analysis are briefly described.

Data-items and spellings

Estes (1993) proceeds with his statistical analysis based on Ebbell's English translation (1973), but it is better to use Egyptian terms as data-items in the construction of the database and the subsequent analyses because the exact meanings of most of the terms remain uncertain and unidentified. Nevertheless, difficulties appear in dealing with the Egyptian terms. The facsimile of the Ebers papyrus in its original Hieratic texts was published by Ebers in 1875. The primary transcription into Hieroglyphic script was provided in works of Wreszinski (1913) and the *Grundriss* (1954–73). There are some minor differences in their choice of signs, but noticeable differences often occur, for instance, in the recognition of *t* and *r* that have a similar hieratic form.

The considerable variation in spellings can bring certain difficulties. The spellings vary in the choice of determinative, the use of alternative or substitution of signs, in the position of signs and sometimes in gender and in the use of a singular or plural form. Mostly, the recognition of the same words spelled differently is clear, and variants in spelling for the same terms can be grouped as one term. Only in some instances, such a classification of terms proves difficult. Attention should be paid to homonyms which, when recognised, are treated separately. Less commonly, terms are represented only by the determinative sign, and since the phonetic values which can be transliterated are not clear, I have chosen to represent such case by the code for the sign from Gardinar's sign-list.

Accommodation to relational schema

Usually a process called normalisation is undertaken in the formation of the relational schema for data-items. This aims to remove statistical errors in repeated measurements of data. In it, several data-sets that have a prime set of data-items serving as dependency (or determinacy) are formulated and linked structurally so that all data-items can gain their proper association with other related data-items.[221] The main data-sets for the Ebers papyrus are the prescription number, the disease, the material, the composition and application method.

The identification of prescriptions can be made based on the pagination of the papyrus marked by the Egyptian scribe (see p. 59). But the numbering by Wreszinski (Eb.1–877) has come to be widely used, and it seems to be suitable for our database to follow Wreszinski's system. But in some cases, improper separation of a prescription occurs. In such cases a joint numbering should be made (e.g. Eb.728–729; Eb.786–787) (Ghalioungui 1987: 186, 201).[222] Also, in several cases, a paragraph which Wreszinski recognised can include several separate prescriptions in a treatment, and this, for our purpose, requires subdivisions of a prescription number (e.g. Eb.68.1, 68.2; Eb.90.1, 90.2).

The disease terms usually occur in the title of a prescription and in the diagnostic texts, and less commonly in other parts (see p. 25-7). The crucial problem is the occasional indication of a prescription by "another" or "another remedy" that will make no sense in the database. In such cases, we may duplicate the data based on data of the previous prescription.

The identification of the words of medicinal materials is generally clear and can easily be taken as data-items. But on rare occasions repeated mentioning of the same material occurs, for instance, in an instruction for a composition method, a referred material is stated in the composition text (*ḥnḳt* ("beer") is mentioned twice in Eb.59). Making a differentiation between actual materials and the condition of materials is also necessary so that conditions for ritual property are not regarded as prescription materials (e.g. the wax used in the fumigation treatment (Eb.795) is specified to be *hby n mnḥ* ("ibis of wax", i.e. ibis-figured wax model). This should not be confused with wax of the bird).

The instructions for composition and application methods usually appear at the end of a prescription text. Commonly, they take a simple, stacked format like *psi wnm* ("boiled and eaten"; e.g. Eb.44), *šmm swr* ("warmed and drunk") and *psi ꜥft sḏr n i꜡dt swr* ("boiled, strained, it remains during the night in the dew and drunk"; Eb.240), but frequently indication is made by "likewise," and, as in the case of "another," duplication of data should be made based on previous prescriptions.

Criteria of data-item and analysis

Gaining an understanding of Egyptian diseases from the medical papyri is difficult, and this is acknowledged by scholars (see p. 29-36). Many terms relating to a disease are unclear to us, and often we do not even know whether such a term represents a pathological condition, a symptom or aetiological entity. In the analyses, we may use such a specific Egyptian disease term as a criterion and test its particular associations with materials or other elements of the prescriptions. But it is often the case that several disease terms appear in one prescription or a disease is described comprehensively with an indication of the afflicted body parts. For instance, *wḫdw* appears together with some other

Sims (1999) and Manly (1994).

[221] For a basic concept of database design, see Howe (2001: 35–79).

[222] Nevertheless, although these prescription texts belong to the same paragraph, these are separate applications in a treatment. Thus in such case, we may still keep Wreszinski's numbering considering that these remedy are essentially separate ones.

1	Recitation	Eb.1–3
2	Internal disease	Eb.4–335
3	Eye disease	Eb.336–431
4	Skin disease	Eb.432–602
5	Extremities	Eb.603–696
6	Miscellanea	Eb.697–782
7	Women disease	Eb.783–853
8	Anatomical information	Eb.854–856
9	Surgical disease	Eb.857–877

Table 7: Ebbell's (1937: 27) classification of the contents of the Ebers papyrus.

disease terms in several combination patterns and occurs in different parts of the body (see p. 32-4). In such an instance, a consideration of both the disease terms and the comprehensive descriptions of disease necessitate setting different criteria according to the objectives of the test.

With regard to the recognition of disease, Badr (1963: 407) notes that about 250 different kinds of diseases can be distinguished in the Egyptian medical papyri, of which the Ebers papyrus enumerates 170. Reeves (1980: 5) notes that Egyptian texts reveal at least 15 distinct diseases of the abdomen, 11 of the bladder, 10 of the rectum and anus, 29 of the eyes, 6 of the ears and 18 of the skin.

Another possible categorization of diseases follows the classification arrangement of clinical matters in the Ebers papyrus itself. This procedure appears most appropriate as it has been done by Egyptians themselves on the basis of their medical understanding. It can also provide broader groups of prescriptions related to a disease and makes it easier to apply statistical approaches. Ebbell (1937) classified the Ebers papyrus into 9 groups (Table 7), and the *Grundriss* provides a far more differentiated classification of 45 groups (Table 8).[223]

Grapow's group appears to be very precise and often a group contains only a few prescriptions. But it is also certain that further detailed classification is applicable, particularly to Group 2, which contains nearly 180 prescriptions and in which different treatments such as evacuation and worm infection and different forms for administration, can be found.

Consideration on setting criteria to the material terms is also important. Primary criteria pertaining to the materials are source, part/product and conditional property. The source terms comprise the name of the plant, animal or mineral. The part/product terms are specific substances taken or produced from the source. In an analysis, we may use the source such as "acacia" or "donkey" as a primary criterion. Or we may use the part/product such as a "seed," "milk" or "honey" as a primary criterion. Also, materials may be defined through a combination of source and part/product criteria. Applying this system leads to a detailed differentiation of materials, and it is useful, for instance, when testing cases of "milk of a cow" and "milk of a woman who has born a male child." Nonetheless, as most of the material terms are not specifically identified, it is rare to achieve definitive recognition of the source or part/product. The Egyptian word *n* ("of") or the position of a term in the material terms may sometimes provide clues from which we can make assumptions, but these are only approximate.

The mechanical recognition of a material from the combination of material terms, however, is problematic. The term *prt*, for instance, is generally translated as "seed" and *šny* as "hair" (of an animal), but the compounded term *prt-šny* is commonly considered to represent a plant name. The term *tꜣ* can be translated as "soil/land," but the term *tꜣ-msḥ* is aptly understood as "*dung* of crocodile" (see p. 40 n. 97) and terms like *šny-tꜣ* (lit. "hair of land"), *spt-tꜣ* (lit. "leaf of land") and *ḥny-tꜣ* (which may be differentiated from another unidentified plant *ḥny*) are taken as plant names (Westendorf 1999: 502, 507). Also, terms like *ns-š* (lit. "tongue of pound") which is regarded as "cuttlebone," and *irt-pt* (lit. "eye of sky") that do not reveal the actual substance have to be dealt with as a single term representing one material (see p. 40).

Another aspect which has to be taken into account is the presence of synonyms among the Egyptian terms. For example, the terms *tꜣ*, *ḥs*, *ꜣs*, *kꜣyt* and *šꜣw* that are translated as "excrement", "stool", "dung" or "faeces" may all be grouped into a single translation. Further detailed differentiation of the material can be made according to the condition of the material such as *wꜣḏ* ("fresh"), *ꜥnḫ* ("fresh" or "raw"?), "from Upper Egypt" or "from the

[223] Ebers (1875) recognized 37 sections in the Ebers papyrus. As early as 1908, Oefele (1908: 16–17) classified the Ebers papyrus into 45 sections. Bardinet (1995: 157) notes "Le Papyrus Ebers réunit des textes de dates et d'origines différentes, que l'on peut répartir en groupes (groupes 1, 2, etc.). Pour le besoins de l'analyse, ces groupes seront divisés en sousgroupes (groupes 1A, 1B, etc.). Comme pour les autres textes médicaux, l'analyse à laquelle nous allons nous livrer porte essentiellement sur l'arrangement des idées et sur la manière dont le rédacteur du papyrus rend compte de la diversité pathologique à laquelle il a affaire," and he makes a classification of the Ebers papyrus into 33 main groups with some subdivisions in them (1995: 588–9).

1	Recitation	Eb.1–3
2	Disease in belly (internal drug)	Eb.4–187 (excl.Eb.104–121, etc)
3	Disease in belly (ointment)	Eb.104–121
4	Prescription introduced by formula "if you examine"	Eb.188–207
5	Treatment for gastric complaint	Eb.208–220 (excl.Eb.219, 220)
6	Treatment of "*ꜥꜣꜥ*-disease"	Eb.219, 220, 221–241
7	Prescription attributed to the invention of gods	Eb.242–247
8	Treatment of head disease	Eb.248–260 (excl.Eb.251)
9	Uses of the "*dgm*-plant"	Eb.251
10	Treatment for urinary complaint	Eb.261–283
11	Treatment for stomach	Eb.284–293
12	Treatment of "*stt*-disease"	Eb.294–300
13	Separate prescriptions unrelated to the preceding	Eb.301–304
14	Treatment of cough	Eb.305–325
15	Treatment of "*gḥw*-disease"	Eb.326–335
16	Treatment of eye disease	Eb.336–431
17	Treatment of bites	Eb.432–436
18	Treatment of "*ḫnsyt*-disease" (ointment)	Eb.437–450
19	Against greying of the hair and eyebrows	Eb.451–463
20	Causing the hair to grow	Eb.464–476
21	Treatment of the liver	Eb.477–481
22	Treatment of burns and stripes	Eb.482–514
23	Treatment of wound	Eb.515–542
24	Treatment of "*ꜣkwt*-disease"	Eb.543–550
25	Treatment of "*bnwt*-disease"	Eb.551–555
26	Treatment of "*šfwt*-swelling"	Eb.556–591
27	A heterogeneous group	Eb.592–597
28	Treatment for pains in the knee and leg	Eb.603–615
29	Disease of the fingers and toes	Eb.616–626
30	Treatment of "*mtw*" (ointment)	Eb.627–696
31	Masticatories for an inflamed tongue	Eb.697–704
32	Cosmetics	Eb.705–738
33	Treatment of the teeth	Eb.739–740
34	A group lacking uniformity	Eb.750–756
35	Treatment of the right side of the body	Eb.757–760
36	Against coryza	Eb.761–763
37	Treatment of ear disease, etc	Eb.764–782
38	Female genitalia and obstetrics	Eb.783–807
39	Female breast and genitalia	Eb.808–830
40	Genital and menstrual disorder	Eb.831–833
41	Genital complaints, galactagogues and neonatal prognosis	Eb.834–839
42	Pesticides and fumigation of house and cloth	Eb.840–853
43	Cardiovascular system	Eb.854–855
44	Book of vessels	Eb.856
45	Book of vessels (2)	Eb.857–877

TABLE 8: GRUNDRISS' CLASSIFICATION OF THE CONTENTS OF THE EBERS PAPYRUS (AFTER GHALIOUNGUI 1987: 4–7).

shore." Dosage indications attached to materials are also included in the data entry.

The composition methods are usually indicated by simple terms like "boil", "grind" and "mix" as well as making things "into one." Sometimes the instructions in a prescription include several steps of a composition process. The final forms of the remedies specified include a pill, a drink, a suppository, an ointment, a fumigation, an inhalation and a pessary. Duplication often occurs for the meaning of phrases in a text of composition and in a text of the application. For instance, a suppository treatment can be indicated both by a composition text *iri m mt* ("made into a suppository"; e.g. Eb.8, 162) and by an application text *rḏi m pḥwy* ("place into the anus"; e.g. Eb.144–6).[224] Therefore it is practical to use a translation word to cover the same indications.

[224] Actually, the composition and application text in many suppository prescriptions read: *iri m mt rḏi m pḥwy* ("made into a suppository and put into anus") and this indicates these two expressions are mentioning the same method of application.

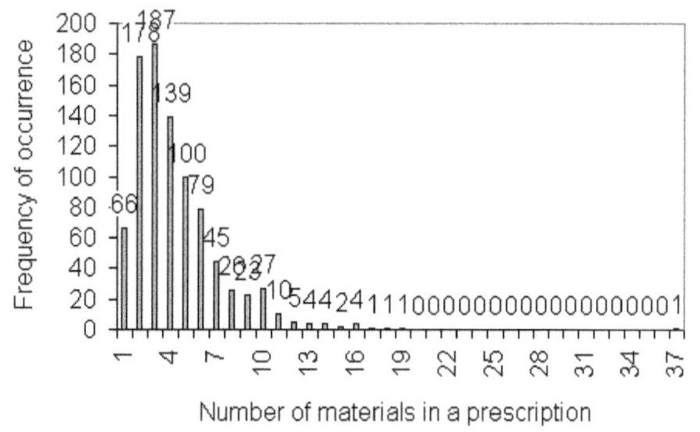

FIG. 11: DIAGRAM SHOWING THE DISTRIBUTION OF NUMBER OF MATERIALS CONTAINED IN A PRESCRIPTION.

Mean	Median	Mode	StDev	Kurtosis	Skewness	Minimum	Maximum
4.40	4.00	3.00	3.01	17.19	2.68	1.00	37.00

TABLE 9: STATISTICAL SUMMARY ON NUMBER OF MATERIALS IN EACH PRESCRIPTION OF EBERS PAPYRUS.

7.2 Testing the hypotheses of Kent Weeks: selected analyses and commentaries

The way in which Egyptian words are regarded and grouped makes a particular difference in the formation of data-items and the structure of the database.[225] This in turn affects the results of the analysis. The data-items and data-sets used in the present work are provided in PDF format contained in the attached CD-Rom.[226] In the following, a selection of statistical analyses are presented and commentary on the findings is provided.

a) Sequence of remedies and number of material

Weeks (1976–78) presents several hypotheses, one of which concerns the relationship between the number of materials in a prescription and the place of a prescription in a group of remedies. He states (1976–78: 295):

> Hermann Grapow arranged the 877 prescriptions in P.Ebers into thirty-seven groups. These groups were defined by their subject-matter, i.e., by the disease they sought to treat, and by the occurrence of such phrases as "The Beginning of Treatment for ..." preceding a group of prescriptions otherwise without such introductory phrases. (These boundaries are fairly certain in about twenty-five of the thirty-seven cases.) Almost without exception, the orthographic variants we have examined distribute themselves in near-perfect correlation with these prescription groupings.

Weeks' preliminary examination of the distribution of orthographical variants leads him to suggest that there were twenty-five to thirty earlier sources of the Ebers papyrus. He continues (1976–78: 296):

> We have said that there are about thirty such groups. They contain an average of twenty-five prescriptions each. The first prescriptions in any of these are generally short ones, containing only three or four drugs. These drugs are usually administered in relatively small quantities. Later prescriptions in the group tend to contain a larger number of drugs—a few contains as many as thirty—and often the quantities of drugs also are increased ... This ordering suggests that an Egyptian physician, after diagnosing a disorder, would have begun his treatment with relatively small doses of a few drugs. If these simple methods failed, he then turn to larger doses and more complex prescriptions

The present database, which aims at simplicity of structure, is not designed to analyse the distribution of orthographical variants, although it is technically possible. But since Weeks was able to point out the close association between a specific group of prescriptions identified by Grapow mainly by the phrase "The Beginning of ..." and the group of orthographical variants, it is possible to test his hypothesis based on Grapow's grouping.[227]

Before testing Weeks' hypothesis, certain conditions must be established. The analysis of the number of materials contained in each prescription reveals a high concentration of prescriptions within the range of lower numbers of materials, and the chance of the occurrence of prescriptions using more than 10 materials is very low (Fig. 11; Table 9). On the basis of this result, it is unrealistic

[225] The structure of a relational database would differ according to the classification of the data-set made through a process called normalisation.

[226] For the contents of the CD-Rom, see the Table of Contents.

[227] There are thirty-seven occurrences of the phrase "The Beginning of ..." in the Ebers papyrus (Eb.4, 104, 221, 242, 261, 284, 294, 305, 326, 336, 437, 451, 464, 477, 482, 515, 543, 551, 556, 592, 603, 616, 627, 697, 705, 739, 750, 757, 761, 764, 783, 808, 840, 854); See Table 8 (p. 76); The thirty-seven group that Weeks mentions as the classification by Grapow might refer to 37 prescription groups out of 45 groupings in the *Grundriss* that start with "The Beginning of ..."

to assume that a group which consists of a large number of prescriptions will exhibit the continuous increase in the number of materials that corresponds to the sequence of the prescriptions. Group 2 (Eb.4–184), for instance, contains about 180 prescriptions.[228] Thus the conditions for testing the hypothesis will be (1) to check if the group starts with the smallest number of materials in the group and (2) to undertake a correlation test between the number of materials and the prescription number with only limited small number of prescriptions from the first prescription of the group.

The number of materials used in the first prescription of Group 2 (Eb.4) is 2, which is not the smallest one in the group. But among these 180 prescriptions in this group, there are only 3 prescriptions (Eb.53, 68.2, 180) that use a single material, and it seems this group starts with a prescription using a smaller number of materials. An increase in the number of materials for the first 10 prescriptions is noticeable (Table 10), and actually a correlation test can indicate its high correlation (r = 0.781), and the probability value derived can also confirm its significance (p = 0.007).[229]

Eb.4	2
Eb.5	3
Eb.6	3
Eb.7	3
Eb.8	3
Eb.9	4
Eb.10	4
Eb.11	5
Eb.12	3
Eb.13	6
Eb.14	3
Eb.15	2
Eb.16	5
Eb.17	6
Eb.18	3
Eb.19	6
Eb.20	3
Eb.21	2
Eb.22	4
Eb.23	10

Table 10: Number of materials of the first 20 prescriptions of Group 2.

However, when we include another 5 prescriptions in the analysis, no significant correlation is indicated (r = 0.420; p = 0.118). The number of materials in the first prescription of Group 3 (Eb.104–121) is 3, with the lowest in this group being 2 which occurs only once (Eb.118). But the correlation test on the first 10 prescriptions denies the significance of the correlation (r = 0.339; p = 0.336). The first 6 prescriptions of Group 6 (Eb.221–241) that start with 4 in number, show a strong correlation (r = 0.882; p = 0.019), though testing with the first 10 denies the significance (r = -0.033; p = 0.926). The 6 prescriptions of Group 7 (Eb.242–247) show no significance in correlation (r = -0.564; p = 0.243). Similarly, the first 10 prescriptions of Group 10 (Eb.261–283) (r = -0.073; p = 0.839) and Group 11 (Eb.284–293) (r = -0.287; p = 0.420) seem to have no correlation. In Group 14 (Eb.305–325), the first 9 prescriptions correlate significantly (r = 0.873; p = 0.002), but the inclusion of the 10th prescription reduces the correlation value (r = 0.536; p = 0.109). The same way of testing on the rest of the Groups brings a negative result in terms of a correlation, except in the case of Group 25 (Eb.551–555) which contains only 5 prescriptions (r = 0.893; p = 0.040), and Group 31 (Eb.697–704) which contains only 8 prescriptions (r = 0.832; p = 0.010), and the first 10 prescriptions of Group 39 (Eb.808–830) (r = 0.763; p = 0.010). It must be noted that the number of materials used in the first prescription in a group is generally less than 4. In 12 groups, the first prescription takes the smallest number of materials, and in 10 groups the first prescription takes the second smallest, and in the other 10 groups it takes the third.

From these results, we may observe that although the first prescription of a group tends to take a smaller number of materials and there are certain cases where the number of materials increases according to the progression in the sequence of the prescriptions, such cases seem to be limited to some particular small set of prescriptions, and they cannot be interpreted as a general trend of a system underlying the Ebers papyrus. We may conclude that there is no general correlation between the number of materials and the position of a prescription in the sequence of a group, and therefore we may discard this hypothesis.

Nonetheless, it is noteworthy to mention that the practice of treatment initiated by applying a weaker drug and then proceeding to the application of stronger medicine is common both in herbal and modern medicine. But one must bear in mind that the degree of efficacy and potency of a remedy is not necessarily related to the number of materials or their doses (see p. 65 n. 200).

b) The material of vehicles and their place in prescriptions

In his study, Weeks (1976–78: 297) made the following observation:

[228] In this section, the prescription group number refers to that of the *Grundriss*, see Table 8 (p. 76).

[229] The correlation value (r) is between -1 and +1. A correlation of + 1 means that all of the data points fall perfectly on a line of positive slope. The correlation near 0 means weak linear relationship. Probability (p-value) is compared to determine if one should accept or reject a hypothesis. Commonly the 0.05 cut-off is used, but infrequently, the 0.01 cut-off is used. If the probability level is less than 0.05 then one must reject the null hypothesis (i.e. that there is no statistically significant difference between the groups being studied); For a basic concept of correlation test and p-value, see Sims (1999: 23–24, 51); Figures are derived by Excel with StatPlus add-in.

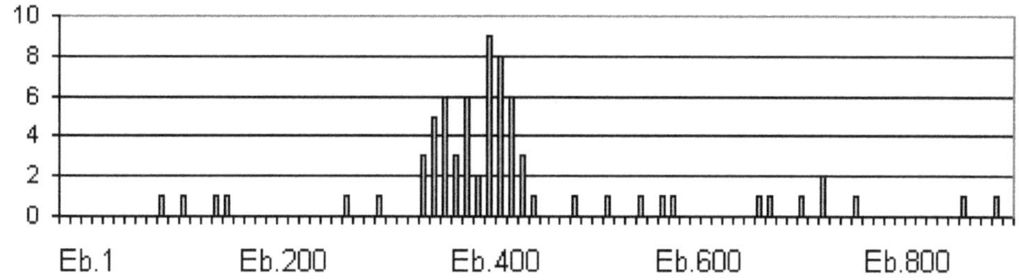

FIG. 12: DISTRIBUTION OF *msdmt* IN THE EBERS PAPYRUS (BIN = 10).

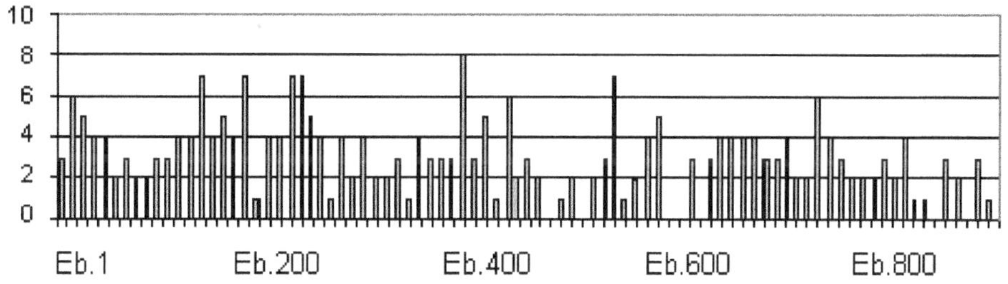

FIG. 13: DISTRIBUTION OF *bit* IN THE EBERS PAPYRUS (BIN = 10).

> There is a tendency in most of the Ebers prescriptions to arrange the drugs in a hierarchical order: the principal ingredients are listed toward the beginning of a prescription, less important drugs follow, and any liquid medium used to facilitate ingestion or application is given last.

This hypothesis is difficult to examine since it is not easy for us to establish whether a material is a principal ingredient according to ancient Egyptian pharmacological ideas. A measurement of the significance of a material may be determined through examining the specific association of a material to a particular Group (i.e. a clinical matter). A material called *msdmt*, which is identified as stibium or galena, is known as a common ingredient for eye cosmetics in ancient Egypt. The distribution pattern of this material in the Ebers papyrus shows its high concentration in the section on eye remedies (Eb.336–431) (Fig. 12), and actually, 52 out of the 72 times of its total occurrence (72.2%), *msdmt* is involved in 96 prescriptions of Group 16.

In the 52 eye remedies that employ *msdmt*, this material is listed in first position 26 times (50%), in second position 15 times (28.8%) and in third position 6 times (11.5%). Another material called *snn* exhibits a strong relationship with *msdmt*. This material occurs only 14 times in the Ebers papyrus, but 12 occurrences appear in the 52 eye remedies that include *msdmt*.[230] In these remedies *snn* takes the first position only once, and is mostly listed in the middle. By contrast, *bit* ("honey"), which can serve as vehicle for a remedy, tends to appear at the end of the lists. In 52 eye remedies with *msdmt*, *bit* is employed in 18 cases, and appears at the end in 13 cases.

Among 505 material words used in the Ebers papyrus, *bit* has the highest frequency of occurrence (268 times), and it is widely distributed throughout the papyrus (Fig. 13).

In 129 out of the 268 occurrences of *bit* (48.1%), it is listed at the end, in 64 (22.7%) in second position from the end, and in 41 (15.2%) it is third from the end; but only in 26 (9.7%) does it occur in the first position (in 4 there is only 1 material; but 5 cases contain 8 to 16 materials). A similar tendency can be found with other substances that are liquid mediums. Thus *irp* ("wine") is listed at the end in 19 of 41 cases (46.3%) and appears second from the end in 7 of 41 cases (17%), while it appears in first position in only 4 of 41 cases (9.7%). The material *ḥnḳt* ("beer") takes the last position in 96 of 126 cases (76.1%) and second from the end in 13 of 126 cases (10.3%), while only in 5 of 126 cases (3.9%) is it assigned to the first position. For *mw* ("water" or watery substance taken from a material), 104 of 136 cases (76.4%) are listed at the end and 17 of 136cases (12.5%) appear second from the end; but in 15 of 136 cases (11%) it takes the first position and in 6 cases it is the only material.

There are certainly cases that show an overlap for some liquid mediums in a prescription. There are 28 cases of overlap of *bit* and *ḥnḳt*, and *ḥnḳt* comes before *bit* in 8 instances. In 39 prescriptions *bit* and *mw* appear together, and in 9 cases *mw* comes before *bit*. In 18 prescriptions *bit* and *irp* are combined, and in 7 cases *irp* comes before *bit*. Only two prescriptions (Eb.136, 151) contain these three materials at the same time. The notable feature is that since these materials tend to occur in the later part of a

[230] Eb.260 also shows the combination of *snn* and *msdmt*.

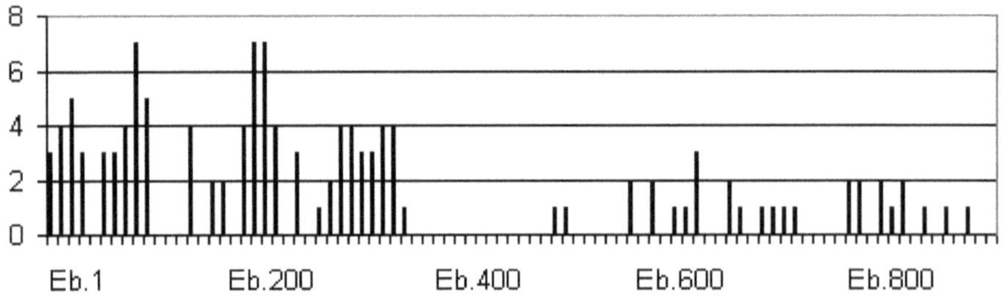

FIG. 14: DISTRIBUTION OF *ḥnḳt* IN EBERS PAPYRUS (BIN = 10).

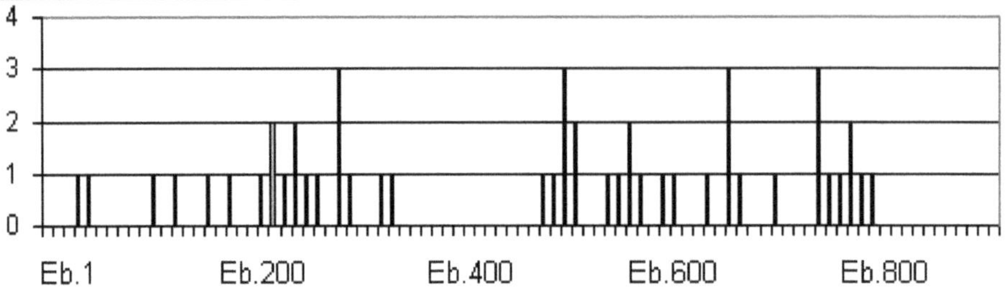

FIG. 15: DISTRIBUTION OF *ḳmyt* IN EBERS PAPYRUS (BIN = 10).

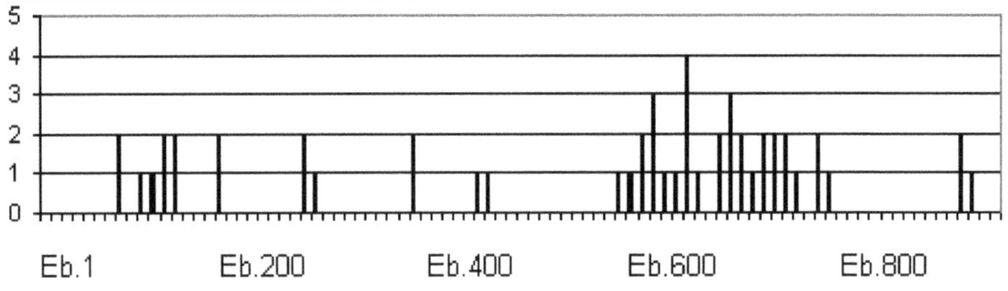

FIG. 16: DISTRIBUTION OF *ḥsmn* THROUGHOUT EBERS PAPYRUS (BIN = 10).

prescription, when they are included in a prescription they tend to appear side by side (60.7% for *bit* and *ḥnḳt*; 72.2% for *bit* and *mw*; 50% for *bit* and *irp*).

From these facts we may confirm that the vehicle materials are listed in the last part of a prescription. The trend for the position of *msdmt* and *snn* in eye-remedies may indicate that the principal substance tends to be written down in first position in the prescription, although there may be a problem identifying *msdmt* as a principal ingredient of an eye prescription purely from its high frequency of occurrence in the eye remedy section.

Nevertheless, it seems it is difficult to apply the same method of measuring significance of function in prescriptions to the other materials because the distribution patterns of other materials seldom show a particular feature or such a clear indication as in the case of *msdmt*, although some materials do form specific distribution patterns. The distribution pattern of *ḥnḳt* shows its strong association with remedies for internal diseases (Fig. 14), and in fact 76.1% (96/126) of its occurrences appear in the second group of Ebbell's classification (Eb.4–335) (see Table 7).

Also, the distribution pattern of *ḳmyt* ("gum") could be interpreted as indicating a tendency towards avoiding its usage in eye remedies (0 in Group 16) (Fig. 15).

The material *ḥsmn* ("natron") seems to have a strong association with skin disorders (Fig. 16).

Other materials that appear to show a certain indicative pattern could be *bnr*, *ḥmꜣt*, *hꜥs*, *mnḥ*, *sꜥm*, *šꜥw*, *sskꜣ*, *swt*, and *tꜣḥt*.[231]

c) Arrangement and combination of materials

Another hypothesis put forward by Weeks (1976–78: 297) is that:

> The arrangement and combination of drugs in P.Ebers suggest that drugs were systematically applied in the treatment of medical disorders by persons whose knowledge of materia medica was more sophisticated than some writers on ancient medicine have previously thought.

[231] See CD-Rom: 14) TermFrqCht.pdf and 15) MateFrqCht.pdf.

This hypothesis is what we are most interested in, but it is obviously the most difficult one to examine. This is principally because, unlike a simple system of listing prescriptions according to the number of materials or unlike the rule of putting vehicle materials at the end in a prescription, the pharmacological system is, in general, much more complicated. The observation of a specific combination, its location of distribution and frequency ratio does not necessarily lead to the conclusion about the presence of a pharmacological system. Also, related to the complexity of pharmacological theory is the fact that specific patterns revealed through an analysis are difficult to understand from a pharmacological perspective.

Analyses reveal that most materials involved in the Ebers prescriptions have a low frequency of occurrence. There are, according to the classification of material terms undertaken in the current study, 505 terms used to represent the source or part/product of a material. These terms make a total of 5057 occurrences of materials throughout the Ebers prescriptions. The materials that have the higher frequency seem mostly to be the materials used as vehicles including *bit* (268 times), *mrḥt* ("oil" or "fat") (208), *mw* (136) and *ḥnḳt* (126) (Table 11).

There are only 19 terms (3.7% of the word list) which occur more than 50 times, but they occupy 38.7% (1960/5057) of the total occurrence of materials. 33 terms (6.5% of the word list) that appear more than 40 times occupy nearly half of the total occurrence (50.7%; 2567/5057). In contrast, 178 terms (35.2% of the word list) occur only once. As many as 400 materials (79.2% of the word list) appear no more than 10 times, but they form 22.5% (1138/5057) of the total occurrences.[232]

Analysing this situation, with precise recognition of materials made through the combination of source and part/product terms, yields a similar result. From the combinations among 505 material terms, a differentiation of 715 materials can be made. These 715 materials make a total of 3987 cases of occurrence throughout the Ebers prescriptions. Only 19 materials (2.6% of detailed material list[233]) with a frequency of more than 40 occupy 37.0% (1478/3987) of the total, and 391 materials (54.6% of detailed word list) appear only once, occupying less than 10% (9.8%; 391/3987) of the total.[234] A similar situation is observed in the particular analyses when specific materials are recognised by the further addition of conditional properties, thereby creating 872 separate materials.

These facts indicate that there are a few materials repeated frequently, but the majority of the materials have a very low frequency of occurrence. Consequently, we cannot expect to have a high frequency of the specific combinations of most of the materials, and this fact is confirmed by testing the frequencies of combination patterns for the materials.

Table 12 is a cross-tabulation showing the combinations among the 19 materials (recognised with source and part/product) that have a frequency of more than 40, that occur in 406 prescriptions that have at least 1 combination among these materials.[235] The materials *bit* and *mrḥt* that have a high frequency (249 and 150 respectively) in the material list appear in these 406 prescriptions (186 and 96 times), but there are only 38 cases where they appear together, and that is the highest figure in this test.

1	*bit*	268
2	*mrḥt*	208
3	*mw*	136
4	*prt*	132
5	*ḏꜣrt*	127
6	*ḥnḳt*	126
7	*snṯr*	118
8	*dḳr*	110
9	*ꜥḏ*	105
10	*ḥmꜣt*	87
11	*msdmt*	72
12	*sṯy*	71
13	(E1)	71
14	*bnr*	61
15	*irtt*	57
16	*wꜥn*	55
17	*ḥsmn*	53
18	*ḏrḏ*	53
19	*ꜥntiw*	50
20	*ḳmyt*	49
21	*dꜣb*	48
22	*ḥsꜣ*	47
23	*šndt*	47
24	*giw*	46
25	*mnḥ*	44
26	*prt-sni*	42
27	(G38)	42
28	*tpnn*	41
29	*irp*	41
30	*wꜣḏw*	40
31	*mnšt*	40
32	*šni-tꜣ*	40
33	*išd*	40

Table 11: Material terms and their frequency > 40*

*A code inside a bracket, such as (E1) and (G38), refers to the code of Gardiner's sign list.

[232] See CD-Rom: 07) TermFrqSort.pdf.

[233] See CD-Rom: 03) TermAssoc.pdf and 04) MatePre.pdf.

[234] See CD-Rom: 08) MateFrqSort.pdf.

[235] Except for *prt-wꜥn*, the materials appear to be represented by one single term, but these are actually materials that occur in the list of materials represented through the combination of source and part/product. Due to this factor, some figures of the frequency ratio differ from the descriptions in the previous part of this study.

	Total	*ʿntiw*	*bit*	*ḏ3rt*	*ḥm3t*	*ḥnḳt*	*ḥsmn*	*mnḥ*	*mrḥt*	*msdmt*	*mw*	*prt-sni*	*snṯr*	*d3b*	*mnšt*	*prt- wʿn*	*ḳmyt*	*šni-t3*	*šty*	*tpnn*
ʿntiw	**38**	—	11	4	4	2	3	8	7	10	2	8	18	0	1	6	1	2	6	5
bit	**186**	11	—	30	26	23	14	15	38	17	26	20	28	15	10	17	13	25	27	11
ḏ3rt	**88**	4	30	—	12	13	7	9	22	9	18	3	18	8	8	3	7	5	11	9
ḥm3t	**74**	4	26	12	—	9	22	6	23	3	3	4	17	2	8	3	5	2	6	6
ḥnḳt	**75**	2	23	13	9	—	0	0	7	0	4	7	16	23	3	16	1	14	3	11
ḥsmn	**44**	3	14	7	22	0	—	1	17	4	1	4	8	2	6	1	2	3	8	3
mnḥ	**38**	8	15	9	6	0	1	—	14	4	3	3	12	1	3	3	5	0	4	5
mrḥt	**96**	7	38	22	23	7	17	14	—	6	6	7	14	2	5	5	3	3	9	6
msdmt	**53**	10	17	9	3	0	4	4	6	—	10	3	11	0	12	0	0	1	12	2
mw	**77**	2	26	18	3	4	1	3	6	10	—	7	11	15	0	7	13	0	23	2
prt-sni	**38**	8	20	3	4	7	4	3	7	3	7	—	9	5	1	6	3	3	6	4
snṯr	**94**	18	28	18	17	16	8	12	14	11	11	9	—	20	6	22	7	6	22	19
d3b	**48**	0	15	8	2	23	2	1	2	0	15	5	20	—	1	13	7	6	16	15
mnšt	**34**	1	10	8	8	3	6	3	5	12	0	1	6	1	—	0	4	1	9	2
prt- wʿn	**41**	6	17	3	3	16	1	3	5	0	7	6	22	13	0	—	2	4	6	14
ḳmyt	**32**	1	13	7	5	1	2	5	3	0	13	3	7	7	4	2	—	0	13	1
šni-t3	**36**	2	25	5	2	14	3	0	3	1	0	3	6	6	1	4	0	—	2	4
sty	**68**	6	27	11	6	3	8	4	9	12	23	6	22	16	9	6	13	2	—	5
tpnn	**38**	5	11	9	6	11	3	5	6	2	2	4	19	15	2	14	1	4	5	—

TABLE 12: CROSS-TABULATION: THE COMBINATION OF MATERIALS.

The material *mrḥt*, which is commonly translated as "oil" or "fat" and which can be a vehicle material, occurs 96 times in the set of 406 prescriptions. Although this material is actually the material with the second highest frequency in the list of material terms (208) (see Table 11), the differentiation of this material through the combination of its source reduces the frequency of each specific *mrḥt* material. This material can be characterised more precisely by 21 terms that specify its source, including (G38) (22 cases), *db* (9), *miw* (4), *ḥf3* (4), *ꜥpnnt* (2), *st* (2), *msḥ* (2), (E1) (1), *gnw* (1), *ibṯrsw* (1) *inst* (1)[236], *ꜥdw* (1), *m3iḥs* (1), *trp* (1), *nꜥr* (1), *ni3w* (1), *niw* (1), *pnw* (1), *š3* (1), *swg* (1) and *int* (1) (these combination occur in 59 cases). There may have been a special significance in specifying different sources and differentiating them pharmacologically, but if we simply regard *mrḥt* as a vehicle material such differentiation would not make sense. So, we may set a special criterion of *mrḥt* to which all kinds of *mrḥt* materials are assigned, and this may bring about a different description from above.[237] However, there are cases that may infer the significance of recognising materials through the combination of source and part/product. A plant called *wꜥn* which is commonly identified as juniper occurs 55 times in the Ebers papyrus, and it mostly takes the *prt* part ("seed" or "fruit") (45 cases; 84%) and other parts including *ḫp3w* (3), *wst* (2), *tp3*wt (1), *ḏꜥꜥ* (1) and *ꜥḏ* (1). When *prt* appears (132 cases) to be taken from a source, the *wꜥn*-plant appears as its chief source (45) followed by *tḥwy* (18), *ḫ3syt* (10), *š3w* (9), *š3ms* (8), *dgm* (7), *ḏ3s* (5), *m3tt* (5), *tnti* (4), *ibw* (3), *s3r* (3), *imst* (2) and others more. In contrast, *ḏ3rt*, an uncertain plant that is assumed to be carob or colocynth, is a plant which occurs with high frequency (127) but it is rarely specified which part is to be used. But in the 33 cases where a part is mentioned, the *prt* part is never taken. Instead, the *dḳr* product that is translated as "powder" and alternatively as "flour" (17) or its *mw* (i.e. fluid substance) (10) are specifically related to this plant. We may notice the significance of the differentiation of *irtt* ("milk") (57) that can be characterised by *mst-ṯ3y* ("a woman who has born a male child") (11) and (E1) ("cow") (11) as well as other sources *rmṯ* (4), *nht* (4), *ꜥ3* (4) and *ḥmt* (1) in a pharmacological perspective because we can assume the Egyptians attributed a special magical property to the milk of a woman who has born a male child (see p. 28).

bit and *mrḥt*	38
bit and *ḏ3rt*	30
bit and *snṯr*	28
bit and *sty*	27
bit and *ḥm3t*	26
bit and *mw*	26
bit and *š3š3*	25
bit and *šni-t3*	25
mw and *sty*	23
bit and *ḥnḳt*	23
ḥm3t and *mrḥt*	23
ḥnḳt and *d3b*	23
snṯr and *sty*	22
snṯr and *prt-wꜥn*	22
išd and *d3b*	22
ḥm3t and *ḥsmn*	22
ḏ3rt and *mrḥt*	21
bit and *prt-sni*	20
snṯr and *d3b*	20
ḥnḳt and *išd*	20
snṯr and *tpnn*	19
ḏ3rt and *snṯr*	18
ꜥntiw and *snṯr*	18
ḏ3rt and *mw*	18
bit and *prt-wꜥn*	17
bit and *msdmt*	17
ḥm3t and *snṯr*	17
ḥsmn and *mrḥt*	17
d3b and *sty*	16
d3b and *wnšy*	16
ḥnḳt and *prt-wꜥn*	16
ḥnḳt and *snṯr*	16
d3b and *tpnn*	15
bit and *d3b*	15
bit and *mnḥ*	15
bit and *irp*	15
mw and *d3b*	15

Table 13: Combination of two materials (frequency > 14).

The systematic analysis of combination patterns among 715 materials that are regarded through the combinations of source and part/product reveals that there are 10,804 occurrences for the combinations of two materials throughout the Ebers prescriptions, and there are 6,391 patterns with a particular combination of two materials (Table 13).[238] There are 30,126 occurrences of combinations of three materials from the 25,626 patterns with specific combinations (Table 14).[239] The frequency of specific

[236] The *inst* is the substance represented as *inst*(2) in the word list. Here the bracket is removed so as not to be confused with the number of frequency.

[237] Another way of setting criterion will be made by grouping words according to the meaning. For example, the term *ꜥḏ* is also understood as oil or fatty material, and it certainly has a high occurrence frequency (105). There may have been a significant difference between *mrḥt* and *ꜥḏ* both in substantial condition and in pharmacological ideas. But in the specification of its source—namely (E1) (29), (G38) (19), *ni3w* (12), *ꜥš* (9), *ꜥ3* (1), *wꜥt* (1), *wꜥn* (1), *šs3w* (1), *sri* (1), *š3w* (1), *š3* (1), *ḳm3wt* (1), *k3* (1), *gnn* (1) and *ḏd3* (1)—we find some overlaps with the sources of *mrḥt*. If we set a criterion such as "oil" or "fat," it may be possible to deal with *mrḥt* and *ꜥḏ* as essentially the same material.

[238] See CD-Rom: 10) 2MateCombi.pdf.

[239] See CD-Rom: 11) 3MateCombi.pdf; The figures in this section are derived through the purely mechanical operation by programming a cord. They include errors caused by several factors including that the same materials are differentiated only by terms of condition in which they occur in a same prescription, and since the condition terms are not included in this operation, the repetitions are counted. Thus the figures are not quite accurate, though the level of error would not be

ḥnḳt and *snṯr* and *d3b*	14
ḥnḳt and *išd* and *d3b*	14
ḥm3t and *ḥsmn* and *mrḥt*	12
išd and *snṯr* and *d3b*	12
mw and *d3b* and *sty*	11
ḥnḳt and *snṯr* and *prt-wʿn*	11
ḥnḳt and *d3b* and *prt-wʿn*	11
snṯr and *d3b* and *prt-wʿn*	10
snṯr and *prt-wʿn* and *tpnn*	10
bit and *ḥnḳt* and *šni-t3*	10
išd and *d3b* and *tpnn*	10
ḥnḳt and *d3b* and *wnšy*	10
bit and *giw* and *prt-sni*	9
ḥnḳt and *išd* and *tpnn*	9
išd and *mw* and *sty*	9
išd and *d3b* and *sty*	9
išd and *d3b* and *wnšy*	9
ḥnḳt and *išd* and *snṯr*	9
ḥnḳt and *d3b* and *tpnn*	9
mw and *ḳmyt* and *sty*	8
snṯr and *d3b* and *tpnn*	8
snṯr and *d3b* and *wnšy*	8
bit and *m3tt* and *sḫt*	8
bit and *irp* and *šni-t3*	8
bit and *snṯr* and *prt- wʿn*	8
ḥnḳt and *išd* and *prt-wʿn*	8
išd and *snṯr* and *nḳʿwt*	8
m3tt and *sḫt* and *prt-wʿn*	8
m3tt and *sḫt* and *ḫt-ds*	8
išd and *snṯr* and *prt-wʿn*	8
snṯr and *d3b* and *nḳʿwt*	7
snṯr and *d3b* and *sty*	7
bit and *snṯr* and *tpnn*	7
bit and *snṯr* and *sty*	7
bit and *ḥnḳt* and *prt-wʿn*	7
ʿntiw and *giw* and *snṯr*	7
bit and *mw* and *sty*	7
bit and *š3ms* and *š3š3*	7
bit and *ʿḏ*-(G38) and *šni-t3*	7
išd and *d3b* and *prt-wʿn*	7
išd- and *d3b* and *nḳʿwt*	7

TABLE 14: COMBINATIONS OF THREE MATERIALS (FREQUENCY > 6).

combinations does not exceed 38 in the combination of two and 14 in the combination of three materials. A vast number of combination patterns both in the combination of two and three materials are unique to themselves. Technically, it is possible to extract specific combinations for four or five materials, but such an analysis would certainly yield a much lower number for the maximum frequency and produce a large number of unique combination patterns. Nevertheless, specific tendencies can be found including that, with 16 occurrences of the combination of *ḥnḳt* and *snṯr*, *d3b* is associated in 14 occasions, and in 20 cases of the combination of *ḥnḳt* and *išd*, *d3b* also appears 14 times with them. Also, an examination of the location of 12 cases with the combination of *ḥm3t*, *ḥsmn* and *mrḥt* shows that they tend to appear in the section dealing with skin diseases.[240]

A high frequency in the occurrence of particular combinations seems to be related to the frequency of materials in the Ebers prescriptions because the materials that occur with high frequency are more likely to be formed into combinations. But the degree of association between a material and other specific materials can be analysed by measuring the ratio of combination. Just in the case of *snn*, which occurs only 14 times but shows a tendency to be combined with *msdmt* (12 cases with *msdmt* and once with *msdmt-ṯ3y*), this allows us to identify the strong association between a material of even lower frequency with another specific material. Two materials reveal a perfect association with another particular material: in all of its 8 occurrences, *sḫt* appears with *m3tt* (which occurs 28 times), and *ḏrḏ-nbs*, which occurs 5 times, is always combined with *ḏrḏ-šndt* (which occurs 38 times). To a lesser degree *sḫt* also shows association with *prt-wʿn* (which occurs 45 times) in 6 cases and in 5 cases with *bit* (which occurs 249 times). The *š3ms*-plant, which appears 10 times, is associated with *bit* on 9 occasions, and *prt-š3ms*, which appears 8 times, combines 7 times with *bit*. This indicates a significant relationship of *š3ms* with *bit*. Similarly in 10 cases of *mw-ḏ3rt*, it appears with *bit* 8 times, but *dḳr-ḏ3rt* which occurs 17 times shows a lower degree of association with *bit* for they are combined in only 7 cases. Also, the *mm*-plant which occurs 20 times appears with *bit* in 11 cases, and *dḳr-mm* which occurs in 7 times appears with *bit* in 4 cases. The material *sḫpt* occurs 5 times, and it is combined with *snṯr* (which occurs 110 times) in 4 cases. A relatively strong association is found for *bddw-k3* (which occurs 7 times) which is combined 5 times with *ḥm3t* (which occurs 86 times). The material *smt* shows its specific association to five different materials: in 9 of its occurrences, 7 cases combine with *snṯr*, 6 cases combine with *d3b* (which occurs 48 times) and *išd* (which occurs 37 times) and 5 cases combine with *prt-wʿn* and *ḥnḳt* (which occurs 106 times).[241]

The examination of a material's distribution pattern and its association with other materials, as showed above, can certainly reveal the particular trend for the material. But such an approach, limited to one or two materials for analysis, can not be used to illustrate the relationship of a greater number of associated materials. A dendrogram (tree or hierarchical diagram) produced by a clustering algorithm can illustrate the arrangement of the clusters of

significant. The VBA codes used in these analyses are provided in CD-Rom: 18) VBA.pdf.

[240] Eb.115, 119, 120, 246, 547, 550, 571, 588, 634, 663, 689.

[241] See CD-Rom: 05) MateAssoc.pdf.

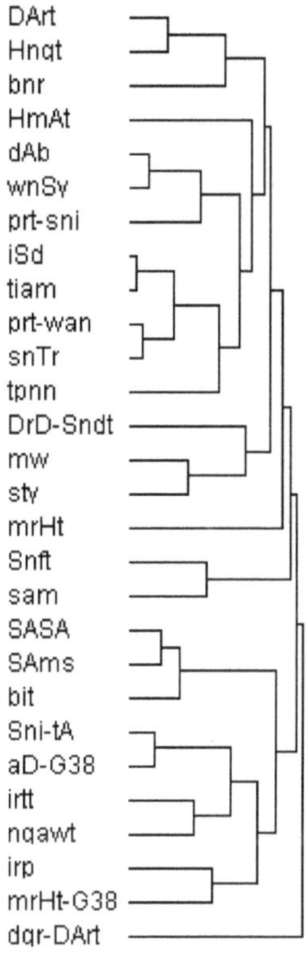

FIG. 17: DENDROGRAM OF MATERIALS IN GROUP 2 (FREQUENCY > 6).

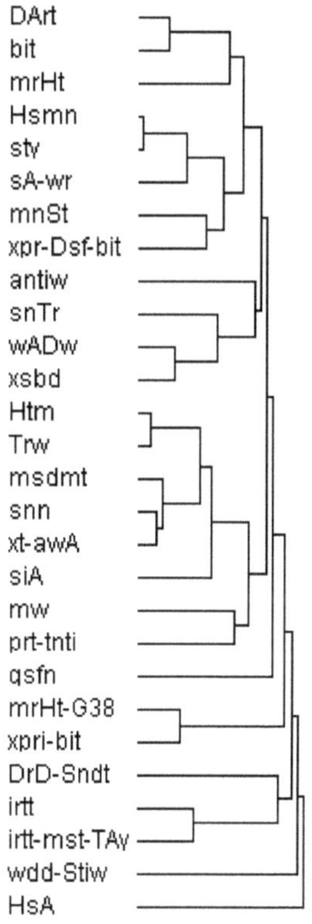

FIG. 18: DENDROGRAM OF MATERIALS IN GROUP 16 (FREQUENCY > 2).

materials.[242] Figures 17 and 18 exhibit the arrangement of materials in Group 2 and Group 16.[243]

The analysis for Group 2 indicates a particular cluster of *išd* and *tiʿm*, and an examination of the location in which it occurs in the Ebers papyrus reveals that this combination is formed only in Group 2.[244] The dendrogram of Group 16 shows a cluster of *ḥsmn* and *sty*, and a characteristic feature of this group is a cluster of *msdmt*, *snn* and *ḫt-ʿwȝ*.[245]

A correspondence analysis can provide us diagrams visualising the arrangement and combination among the materials in a three-dimensional scale.[246] The following diagrams exhibit the associations for materials in Group 2, which mainly contains the prescriptions of internal remedies for diseases in the belly (Fig. 19—due to the length of the diagram, it runs on to the next page).[247]

The three sections of Figure 19 show the three different sides of three-dimensionally represented associations in the analysis. Figure 20 below depicts the same associations in 3D expression.

In the diagram of Figure 18, the degree of association among the materials is indicated by the distance between them and their direction. In this representation, the position of a material which is close to the central axis indicates its mutuality in the relationship with other associated materials. The noticeable associations indicated by the diagram include the relationship between *ḥnḳt* and *bnr*, *tpnn* and *tiʿm*, and *ʿḏ*-(G38) and *irp*. The isolated situation of *ḏrḏ-šndt* and *mrḥt* is also noticeable. The same test applied to Group 16 of eye-remedies reveals the mutual position of *msdmt*, *wȝḏw* ("malachite") and *ḫt-ʿwȝ*, indicating that they are associated with the many materials involved in the analysis (Fig. 21).[248]

As showed in the following figure (Fig. 22), a correspondence analysis can also be run to test the differences between Group 2 and Group 16 in terms of the arrangement of their materials.

In this diagram, the materials that lie at a greater distance from the centre indicate their particularity to a group; and

242 For a basic concept of cluster analysis, see Kachigan (1991: 261–70).

243 The analysis was carried out with Simstat and WordStat; A hieroglyphic transliteration font is not available in these programs, therefore the following letters have been substituted to accommodate this lack: a=ʿ, A=ȝ, D=ḏ, H=ḥ, x=ḫ, X=ẖ, q=ḳ, S=š and T=ṯ.

244 Eb.17, 79, 87, 97, 122.

245 See CD-Rom: 16) Dendg.pdf.

246 For a basic idea of correspondency analysis, see Manly (1994: 201–7) and Le Roux *et al.* (2004: 1–24).

247 The analysis was carried out with Simstat and WordStat.

248 See CD-Rom: 17) CorrAna.pdf.

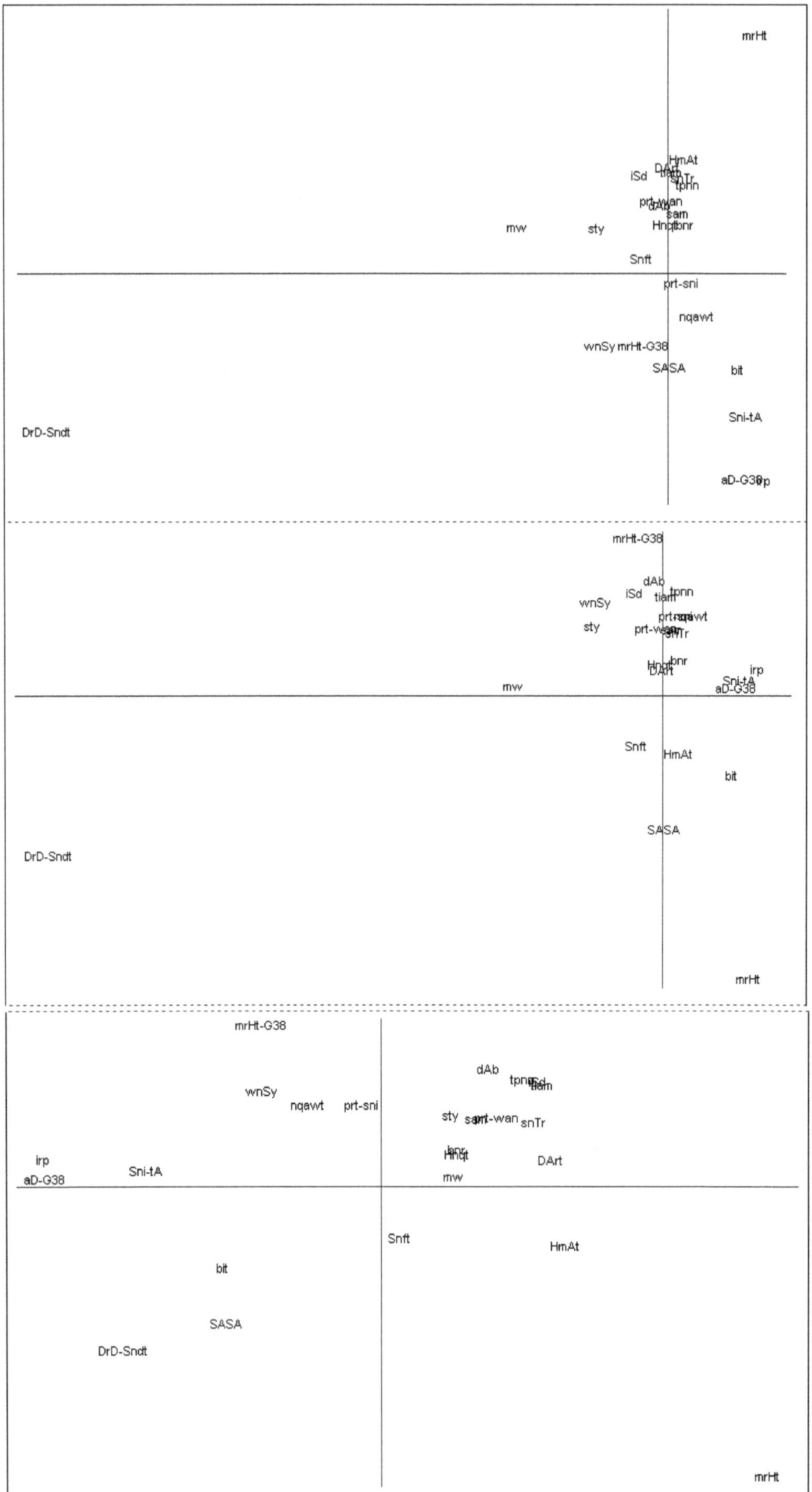

FIG. 19: CORRESPONDENCE ANALYSIS APPLIED TO MATERIALS IN GROUP 2 (FREQUENCY > 7): (TOP: AXIS 1 VS 2; MIDDLE: AXIS 1 VS 2; BOTTOM: AXIS 2 VS 3).

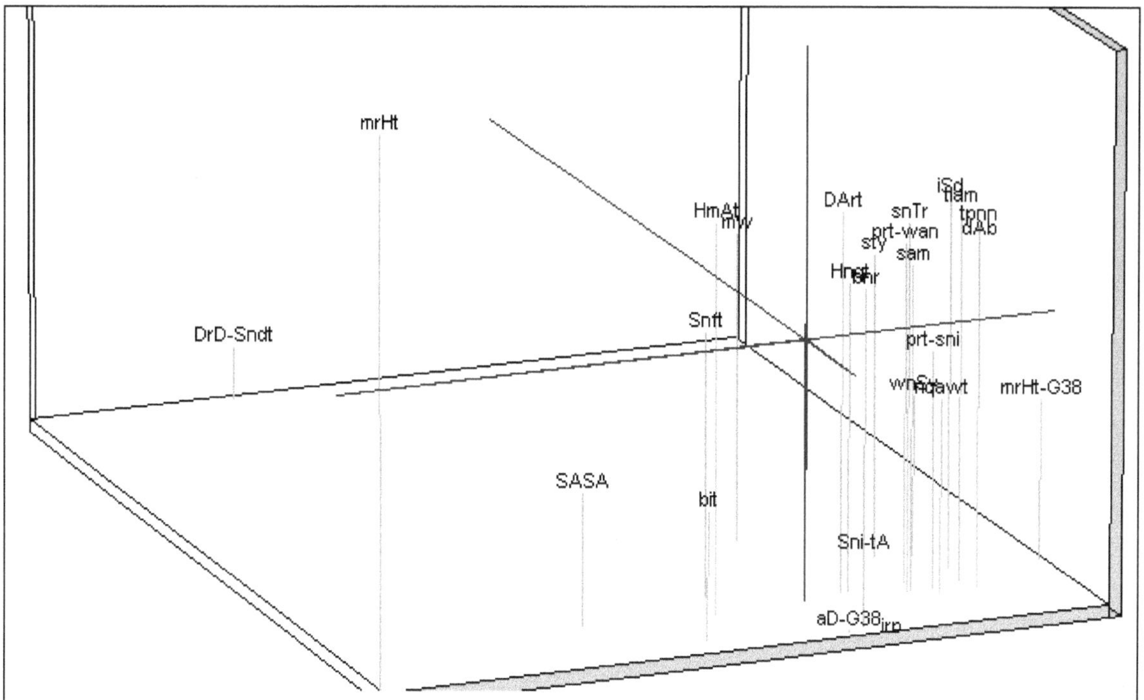

FIG. 20: 3D DIAGRAM: CORRESPONDENCE ANALYSIS APPLIED TO THE MATERIALS IN GROUP 2 (FREQUENCY > 7).

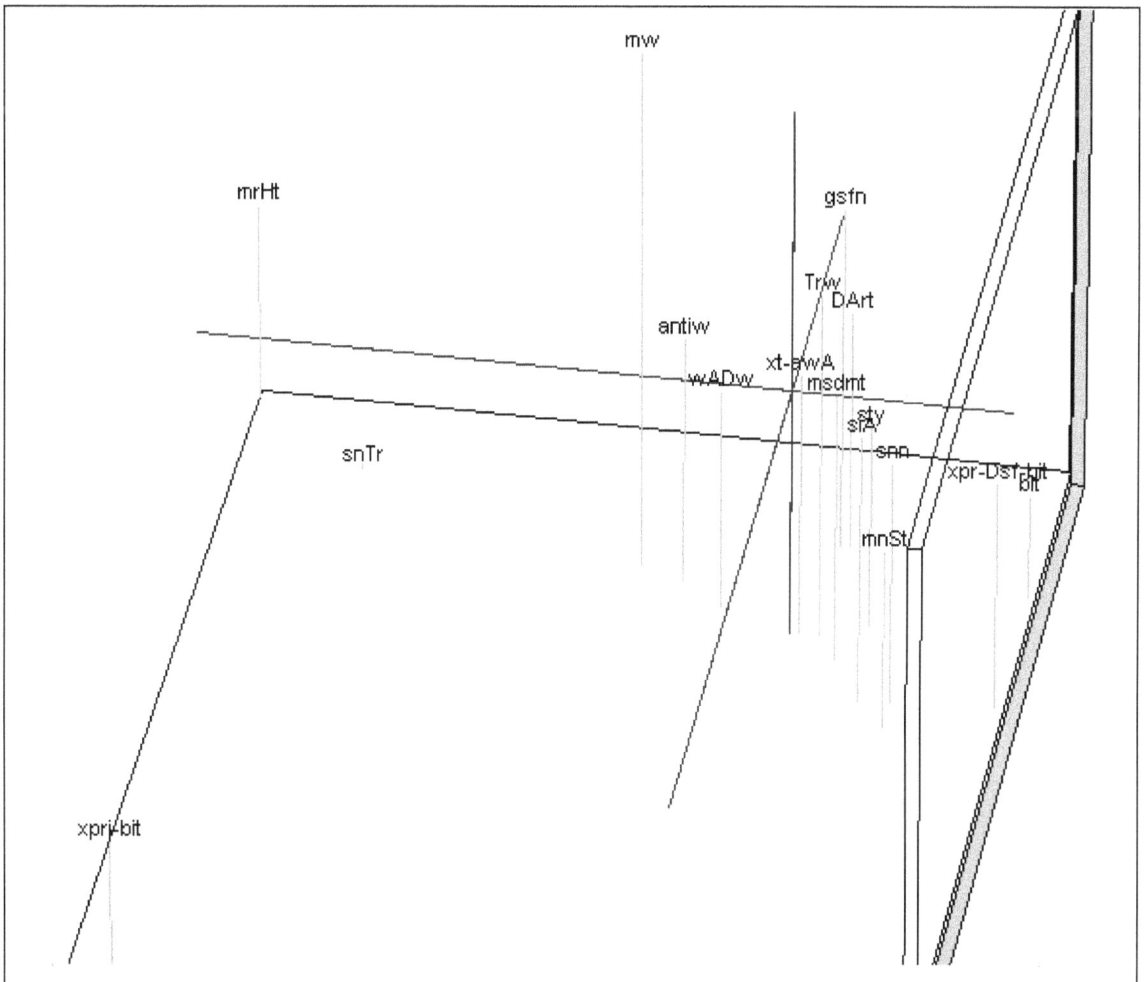

FIG. 21: 3D DIAGRAM: CORRESPONDENCE ANALYSIS APPLIED TO THE MATERIALS IN GROUP 16 (FREQUENCY > 3).

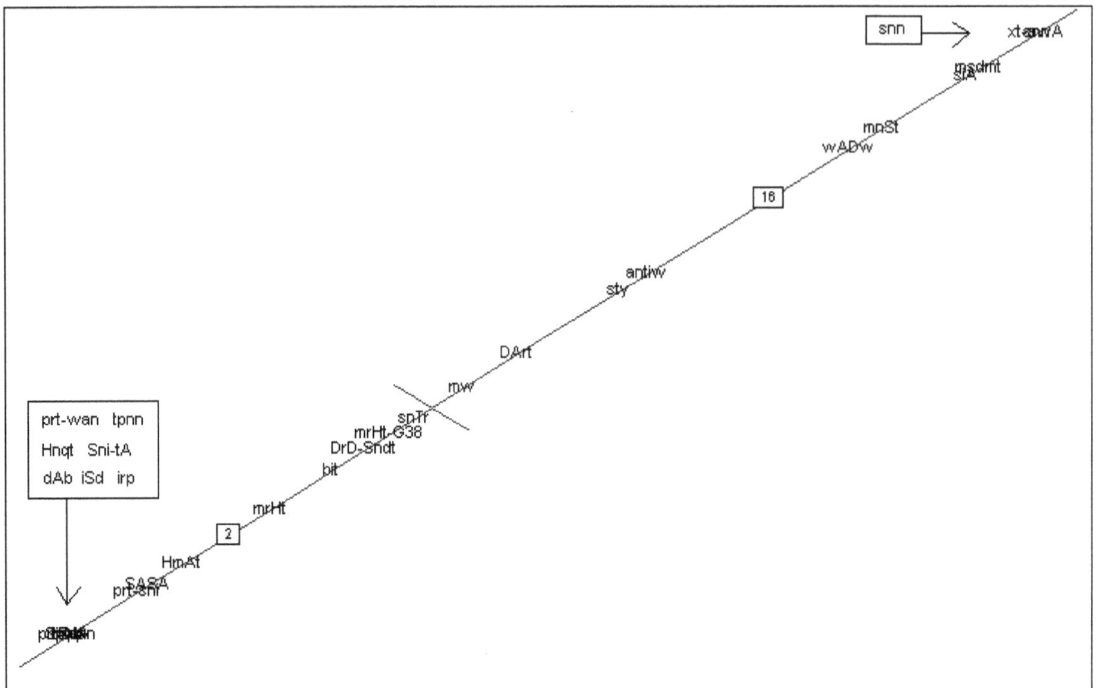

FIG. 22: THE DEGREE OF ASSOCIATION: MATERIALS FROM GROUP 2 AND GROUP 16 (FREQUENCY >10).

the materials near the centre are not characteristic to either group or are equally common to both groups. The diagram shows that *ḫt-ʿw3* and *snn* are particular to eye-remedies (Group 16, top right) and materials such as *ḥnḳt*, *tpnn* and *prt-wʿn* to the treatment of the belly (Group 2, bottom left). It is also possible to include more than two groups into an analysis. The sections of the diagram below (Fig. 23) illustrate the relative positions among Groups 2, 3 (ointment for belly disease), 10 (treatment for urinary complaint), 16 and 23 (treatment of wound).

These diagrams reveal some interesting features: The material *š3š3* has a particularly close association with Group 2; *bnr* and *giw* with Group 10; and *mhḥ* with Group 23. The specifically strong association with belly diseases of materials such as *tpnn*, *tiʿm*, *šni-t3*, *nḳʿwt*, *sʿm* and *šnft*, that form a cluster behind Group 2, is also notable. The Groups 3 and 23, being both mainly remedies of topical application, have a close association particularly through their use of *ʿḏ* and *b3ḳ*. The Groups 2 and 10, both mainly comprising oral remedies, are closely associated in terms of their use of materials such as *ḥnḳt*, *išd*, *prt-wʿn* and *prt-sni*. The diagram also indicates the relatively isolated position of the eye-remedies (Group 16), which means that the prescriptions of this group are distinctly different from the others. The distinctiveness of the eye-prescriptions in the Ebers papyrus can be also showed in a correspondence analysis based on the inclusion of all the groups and materials which appear more than twice (Fig. 24).

The findings revealed by the type of statistical analyses undertaken have their limitations and are of restricted value. The achievement lies only in creating an awareness of characteristics and features. They do not provide us with an interpretation, which would allow us to reach an understanding of the pharmacological principles the prescriptions are based on.

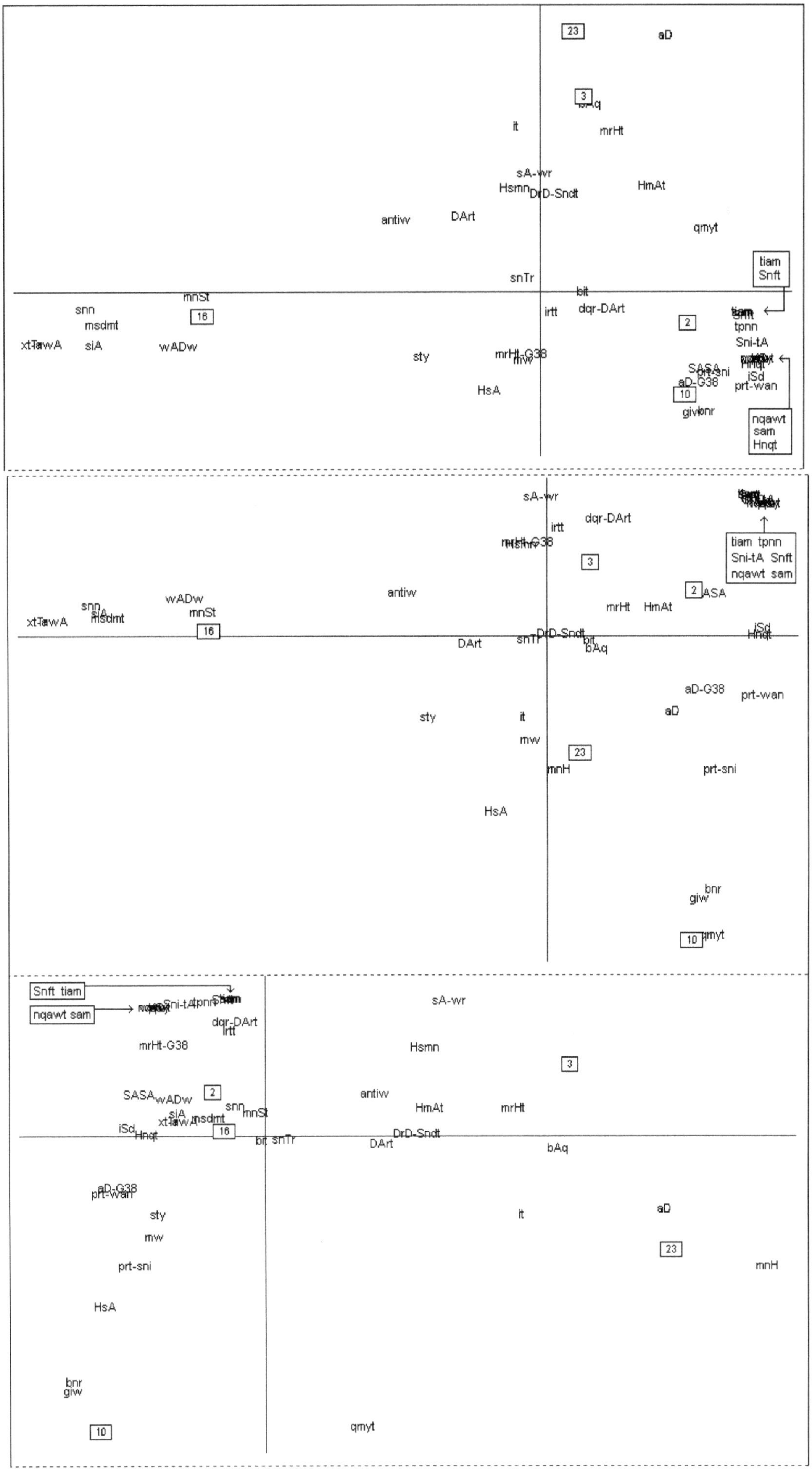
23
aD
3
it
mrHt
sA-wr
Hsmn
DrD-Sndt
HmAt
antiw
DArt
qmyt
tiam
Snft
snTr
mnSt
bit
snn
16
irtt
dqr-DArt
2
msdmt
tpnn
xt-TawA
siA
wADw
Sni-tA
sty
mrHt-G38
SASA
iSd
aD-G38
prt-wan
HsA
10
giw
bnr
nqawt
sam
Hnqt
sA-wr
irtt
dqr-DArt
tiam tpnn
Sni-tA Snft
nqawt sam
3
antiw
2
ASA
wADw
mnSt
mrHt
HmAt
xt-TawA
16
DArt
iSd
Hnqt
bAq
aD-G38
prt-wan
aD
sty
it
mw
23
mnH
prt-sni
HsA
bnr
giw
10
Snft tiam
nqawt sam
sA-wr
dqr-DArt
mrHt-G38
Hsmn
3
SASA
wADw
2
antiw
HmAt
mrHt
snn
mnSt
iSd
16
snTr
DArt
DrD-Sndt
bAq
sty
it
aD
mw
23
mnH
prt-sni
HsA
bnr
giw
10
qmyt

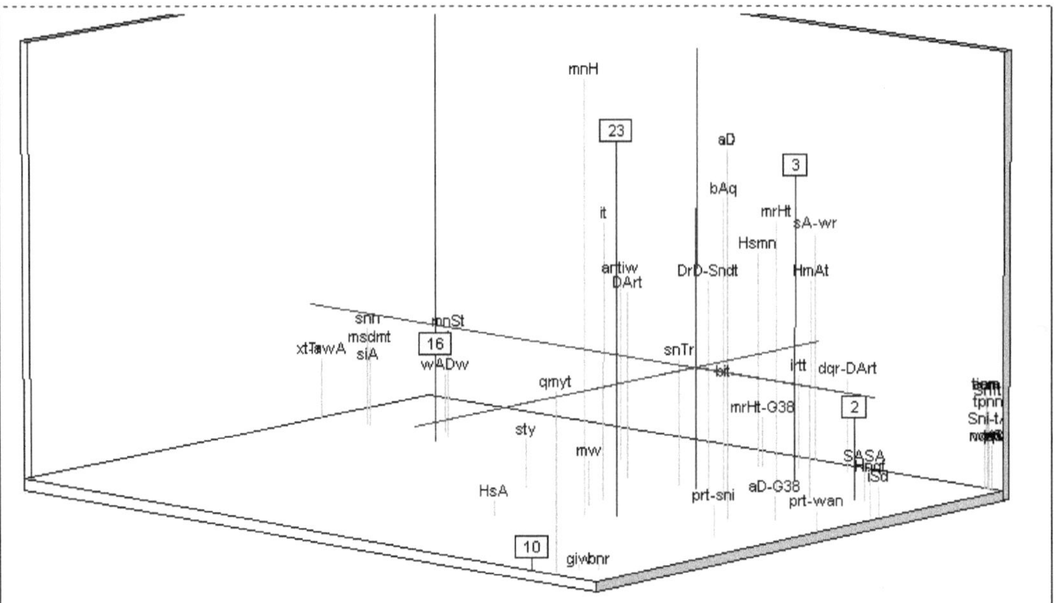

FIG. 23: DIAGRAMS SHOWING ASSOCIATIONS AMONG GROUP 2, 3, 10, 16, 23 IN TERMS OF THEIR ARRANGEMENT AND COMBINATION OF MATERIALS (FREQUENCY>7): (TOP: AXIS 1 VS 2; MIDDLE (UPPER): AXIS 1 VS 2; MIDDLE (LOWER) AXIS 2 VS 3; BOTTOM: 3D).

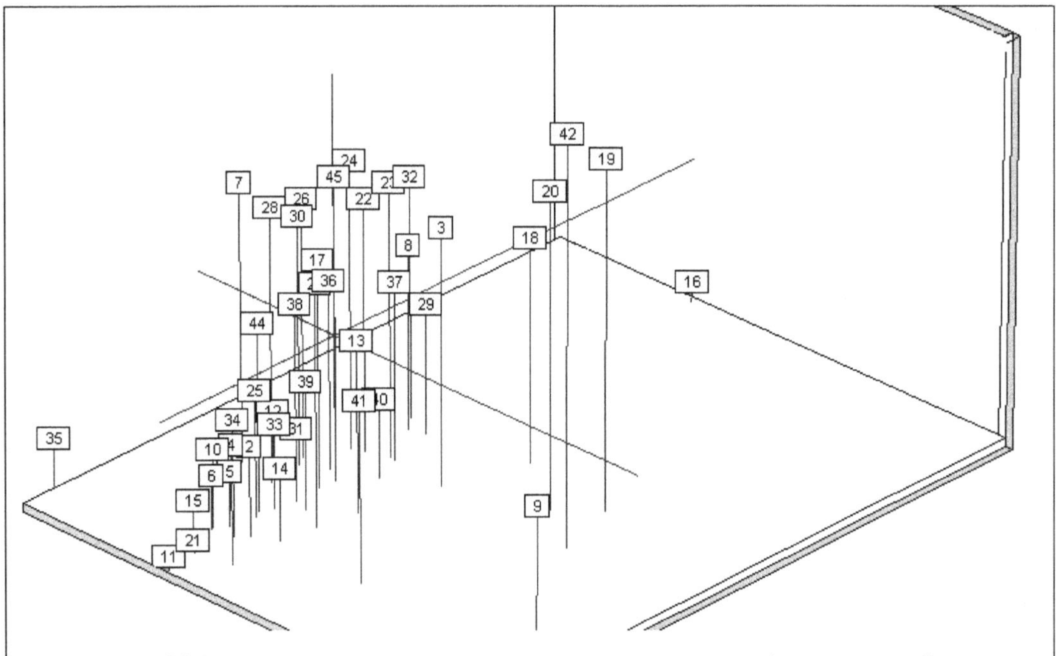

FIG. 24: RELATIVE POSITION IN ASSOCIATION AMONG THE GROUPS (FREQUENCY > 1).

7.3 A special category of prescriptions: said to be designed by six gods

In the Ebers and Hearst papyri (Eb.242–247; He.71–75), there is a set of six prescriptions that—as the text themselves say—have been designed by divinities.[249]

In the Ebers papyrus, the first prescription carries the heading "Beginning of the remedy that Ra prepared for himself." The subsequent 5 prescriptions are marked as the "second," "third" to the "sixth" remedy of this kind. The divinities Shu, Tefnut, Geb, Nut and Isis are each assigned to one of these prescriptions as inventors of the respective remedy for Ra.[250] The most extensive prescription, which is designed by Ra himself, contains as many as 16 materials while the shortest one by Tefnut has only 3 materials. At a

[249] Among the parallel paragraphs contained in the Ebers and Hearst papyri, the first prescription is for some reason missing in the Hearst papyrus.

[250] The second remedy by Shu, however, is mentioned as being designed for himself.

	Eb.242 (Ra)	Eb.243 (Shu)	Eb.244 (Tefnut)	Eb.245 (Geb)	Eb.246 (Nut)	Eb.247 (Isis)
1	*bit*	*dḳr . swt*	*dḳr . ʿmʿʿ*	*dḳr . ḏꜣrt*	*ḏbt*	*prt . šꜣw*
2	*mnḥ*	*ḥmꜣt*	*šnft*	*dḳr . ṯḥwy*	*kfꜣ . ḳꜣdt*	*prt . ḫꜣsyt*
3	*ḫpꜣw . snṯr*	*mrḥt*	*mrḥt* . (G38)	*dḳr . ḫt-ds*	*inr*	*sʿꜣm*
4	*prt . sꜣr*	*dḳr . šꜣw*		*ḫpr-ḏs-f . bniw*	*ḥsmn*	*prt . šꜣms*
5	*. ḏꜣrt*	*ḏʿbt*			*ḥmꜣt*	*prt-sni*
6	*šꜣšꜣ*	*dḳr . ḏꜣrt*			*ꜣḥ*	*bit*
7	*mwt . giw*	*dḳr . iwryt*			*mrḥt*	
8	*prt . ḏꜣs*	*. snṯr*			*ḳmyt*	
9	*ibw*	*ḳstt*			*sft*	
10	*. ḫꜣsyt*	*sty*			*bit* (2)	
11	*ṯḥntt . snṯr*	*ḥsꜣ*				
12	*pršt*					
13	*prt . šꜣw*					
14	*ḫpꜣw . wʿn*					
15	*ḫpꜣw . ʿš*					
16	*ꜣḥ*					

TABLE 15: SIX PRESCRIPTIONS DESIGNED BY DIVINITIES (EB.242–247).

Eb.244 (Tefnut)	Eb.245 (Geb)	Eb.243 (Shu)	Eb.246 (Nut)	Eb.242 (Ra)	Eb.247 (Isis)
	dḳr . ḏꜣrt	*dḳr . ḏꜣrt*		*. ḏꜣrt*	
		ḥmꜣt	*ḥmꜣt*		
mrḥt . (G38)		*mrḥt*	*mrḥt*		
			ꜣḥ	*ꜣḥ*	
				bit	*bit*
		dḳr . šꜣw		*prt . šꜣw*	*prt . šꜣw*

TABLE 16: A SPECIFIC PATTERN OF DUPLICATED MATERIALS IN AN ARRANGED DISTRIBUTION.

glance these prescriptions may appear a random mixture of materials,[251] but actually the characteristic feature of each prescription in terms of the selection of materials is evident. Isis prefers to use the *prt*-part of the plants. Ra uses their *prt*-part and the *ḫpꜣw*-part. But Shu, Tefnut and Geb prefer to take their *dḳr*-part. Nut's remedy may be characterised by its use of mineral substances. We also notice that both the *prt*-part and *dḳr*-part happen to be specified as the *šꜣw*-plant, and the *ḫpꜣw* and *ṯḥnt* parts of *snṯr* are used separately, as if they are different materials in a prescription, while this material can be roughly specified as *snṯr*. In two cases the *dḳr*-part is taken from the *ḏꜣrt*-plant, but in one case the test simply mentions it as the *ḏꜣrt*-plant. A cow is the source of *mrḥt* in one case, but in two cases no specification to *mrḥt* occurs (Table 15).

We can recognise 44 different materials (seen from combinations of source and part/product) in the 6 prescriptions where 50 occurrences of materials can be

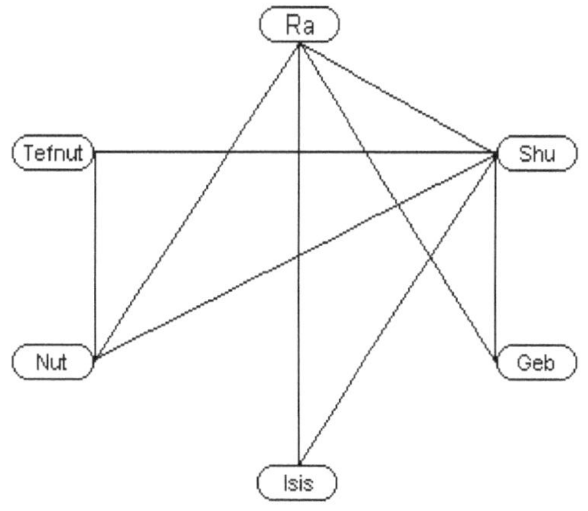

FIG. 25: DUPLICATION PATTERN: REPRESENTED IN THE CONNECTIONS AMONG 6 DIVINITIES.

[251] For Thorwald (1962: 50), the long prescription of Ra is an "apparently random prescription."

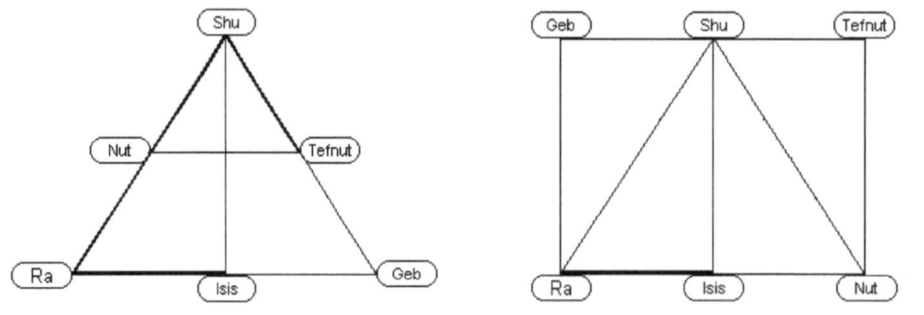

FIG. 26: ALTERNATIVE SYMMETRIC ARRANGEMENTS REPRESENTING THE DUPLICATION PATTERN. THE BOLD LINE REPRESENTS THE OVERLAP OF LINES.

observed. 6 materials appear twice while the rest appear only once. An interesting pattern appears in terms of the distribution of these duplicated materials in that when they are placed so that the same materials are placed side by side, a linear link appears in the arrangement throughout the prescriptions, except that of Tefnut (Table 16).

When we add the materials *ḏ3rt*, *mrḥt*-(G38) and *dḳr-š3w* that are associated with these duplicated materials, as well as the association links of these materials with the deities, we are able to represent the different combinations of three associated deities by a set of four triangles (Fig. 25).

The illustration of this pattern in such an arrangement may, at first glance, not reveal its symmetry. Changes to the positions of the deities can alter the graph into a large triangle or square that bring about a different visual impact (Fig. 26).

There must be an underlying system which leads to a formulation of a pattern, but what the pattern ultimately means remains unclear and impossible to determine at this point in time. We may consider that many of the characteristic features expressed in these six prescriptions are not entirely arbitrary and that they are the result of considerations made by Egyptian physicians against the background of a broad knowledge of medicine. The features of these six prescriptions may express what I choose to call the "dynamics of pharmacology" in ancient Egypt.

7.4 Conclusion and outlook

Our knowledge of ancient Egyptian culture can lead us to the assumption that the Egyptians tended to observe their environment in a logical and systematic way and studies of Egyptian medicine can also confirm this aspect. We may come to think that Egyptian medicine is not a medicine which is understood merely through the "empirico-rational" and "magico-religious" perspectives but also through some other reality beyond these, although yet unknown and hidden.

Through the statistical operations conducted in this current study, the arrangement and combination of the materials in the prescriptions of the Ebers papyrus revealed certain tendencies. Even though the break-through to that hidden reality of the medical principle has not been found, it still remains a possibility that further research should strive to achieve.

Concluding Remarks

A study that investigates the validity of analysing the distribution pattern of materials in the Ebers papyrus involves a range of discussion that often requires quite different areas of expertise such as Egyptian philology, ancient and traditional medicines, modern chemotherapeutic principles, medical history, medical anthropology and statistics as well as database design. This requirement certainly posed difficulties, for as a student of Egyptian archaeology, my accessibility to the expertise of non-Egyptology fields was limited. But it was essential to acquire such special knowledge to be able to participate meaning fully in the discourse related to this subject.

However, after working on all the essential aspects that are necessary for a comprehension of this subject, the question of the methodological validity of a statistical analysis of the pharmacology of the Eber papyrus remains open due to the unusual difficulties of this area of study. In this respect, the present work can be seen as providing a negative report. Yet in reality it is all these hindrances that make this work worthwhile. This is because a proper understanding of the difficulties involved can help identify the limitation to a realistic hypothesis in understanding of the Egyptian medicine, and also it can open up prospects for further study where such a specific problem is dealt with.

The fundamental issue that need to be considered when deciding whether statistical approach to an examination of the Ebers papyrus concerned the quality of the papyrus as a sample body—i.e. a consideration of the fragmentary nature of the medical texts, the possible variations in underlying medical ideas and the medical ideas which persisted in medical traditionalism but more often were modified in the transmission.

The diversity of applicable medical expertise in the interpretation of Egyptian pharmacology is reflected in the many references to Egyptian medicine in the publications of aromatherapy, homeopathy, traditional herbal medicine and even in a recent report of phytochemistry. Thus, a study of Egyptian pharmacology necessitates collaboration with the knowledge of different types of medicine, although it is true that such variation of applicable medical perspectives makes it difficult to have a definitive understanding of Egyptian pharmacology.

The beneficial perspectives gained from incorporating into a study insights gained from different types of medicines derive from the significant historical and cultural "association" shared by them. Studies on herbal medicine note the benefits of a herbal medicine and illustrate a preparation based on old tradition. Publications dealing with traditional systematic medicine explain the theoretical thought that lies behind the attribution of efficacy to herbs and other materials, but they often incorporate modern chemotherapeutic principles to provide a proof of their effectiveness. Works on medical anthropology and medical history analyse the essential cultural thought processes involved in the formation of a medical theory and also reveal the dynamic transmission and complex interaction of medical ideas that occurred in many historical and cultural circumstances. Also, medical pluralism, which exhibits the coexistence of inconsistent medical systems in a culture, and the occasional cases of transmission of a medicine beyond its country and language over one thousand years are a significant feature when considering the background of a medicine.

It was these outlooks that this discussion attempts to incorporate into the discussion because they can provide a helpful perspective for a consideration of the situation of Egyptian medicine. In this study, noticeable is the hypothetical nature of our understanding of Egyptian pharmacology when we base our investigation "empirico-rational" and "magico-religious" principles, but more significant is the observation of the presence of important cultural and medical concepts in ancient Egypt for which we can find parallels in the medicines of other cultures, that also played important roles in these other advanced medicines. It is also significant to note that the transmission of medical knowledge through textual copying in ancient Egypt also find its parallel in the methods used in other cultures.

Study of any patterns in Egyptian prescriptions should be made against the background of the hypothesis that the pattern results from a pharmacological theory. Thus, having a hypothetical understanding of Egyptian pharmacological theory is essential. Although the "empirico-rational" and "magico-religious" perspectives help in assuming the function of an ingredient in a prescription, Egyptian pharmacology can not be defined simply by concepts of medical empiricism or explained by primitive magical and religious belief.

The Egyptians' profound comprehension of medicine can be recognised in their detailed anatomo-physiological and pathological terminology, and in their description of body structure where the function and network of the organs are recognised. The association of such physiological and pathological concepts as *wḫdw*, *stt*, ꜥꜣꜥ and *ḥrrw*-worm is a noticeable indication of the presence of theoretical thought. From comparative study of Egyptian and Greek medicines one can infer the possible presence of an elaborate medical theory in ancient Egypt, based on which the Greeks developed their medicine. With a cross-cultural study of medicines, the presence of parallel cultural components found in ancient Egypt, such as the basic principle of "analogy" and "antithesis" and the concept of universal law, which played an intrinsic role in structuring medical theory in Greece, China and India, is notable. One may argue that the Egyptian approach to the comprehension of nature was rich in the use of logic, and it is not entirely unrealistic to consider that the Egyptians logically incorporated such principles into their medical theory.

The present state of our understanding of Egyptian pharmacology is problematic and insufficient to describe the trend and pattern of the Egyptian prescription. But an important insight may be that it is the poly-pharmacological principle that is needed to illustrate the pattern of Egyptian prescriptions. The study of the principle of poly-pharmacology reveals that different kinds of functions are attributed to each ingredient and that the cooperation of ingredients enhances the efficacy of a remedy; it is this function that the approach via the "empirico-rational" and "magico-religious" perspectives ignore. An irrational or contradictory use of a medicinal material in Egyptian prescriptions is sometimes noted, but it may appear rational when a poly-pharmacological concept, namely the "antago-effect," is applied in the interpretation.

With recent developments in computer-based systematic statistical analysis, it was only a matter of time before this model was used to research the Ebers papyrus. Weeks suggested the validity of this approach some 30 years ago. One can see occasional references made by scholars to pattern in Egyptian prescriptions, and this indicates that attention has been repeatedly paid to the potential of this methodology. Some trends and patterns in the Ebers prescriptions could be extracted from the trial analyses demonstrated in this work, but we are still in the preliminary stage of investigation as far as attempting to set out an interpretation device for the pharmacological meaning of revealed patterns. Hopefully this work will serve as a basis for further investigation in this area of study.

Appendix: Materials identified as Egyptian materia medica[252]

In each category, the materia medica are listed in alphabetical order.

Plant kingdom

Plant names

Acacia (*Acacia nilotica*)(Egyptian: *šnḏt*)	Celery (*Apium graveolens*)	Garlic (*Allium sativum*)	Myrtle (*Myrtus communis*)	Senna (*Cassia angustifolia*)
Acanthus	Cinnamon (*Cinnamonium zeylanicum*) (Egyptian: *ti-šps*)	Grape (*Vitis vinifera*)	Oak (*Quercus robur*)	Sesame (*Sesamum indicum*)
Aloes (*Aloe vera*)	Colocynth (*Citrullus colocynthus*)	Hemp (*Cannabis sativa*)	Olibanum (*gum resin from genus Boswellia*)	Sycamore (*Ficus sycomorus*)
Ammi (*ammi visnaga* / *ammi majus*)	Coriander (*Coriandrum sativum*) (Egyptian: *š3w*)	Indigo (*plant of genus Indigofera*)	Onion (*Allium cepa*)	Tamarisk (*Tamarix nilotica*) (Egyptian: *ỉsr*)
Anise (*Pimpinella anisum*)	Costus	Juniper (*Juniperus phoenicea* / *drupacea*) (Egyptian: *wꜥn*)	Palm	Thyme (*Thymus sibthorpii*)
Asafoetida (*Ferula foetida*)	Cucumber (*Cucumis sativus*)	Leek (*Allium kurrat* / *porrum*) (Egyptian: *ỉ3ḳt*)	Papyrus (*Cyperus papyrus*)	Turpentine
Balanites (*Balanites aegyptiaca*)	Cumin (*Cuminum cyminum*)	Lettuce (*Lactuca virosa*)	Pea (*Pisum sativum*)	Water melon (*Citrullus lanatus*)
Balsam	Cyperus (*Cyperus esculentus*) (Egyptian: *giw*)	Lotus (*Nymphaea lotus*) (Egyptian: *sšn*)	Pine	Weed
Bay	Dill (*Anethum graveolens*)	Manna	Pomegranate (*Punica granatum*) (Egyptian: *inhmn*)	Wheat (*Triticum aestivum*)
Bryonia (*Bryonia dioica*)	Ebony (*Diospyros ebenum*)	Melon (*Cucumis melo*)	Poppy (*Papaver somniferum*)	Willow (*Salix safsaf* / *Salix forrsk*) (Egyptian: *trt*)

[252] The appendix is based on the lists of Egyptian *materia medica* provided by Nunn (1996: 146–61) and Ghalioungui (1973: 141–3), and also with reference to the translation of the Ebers papyrus by Ebbell (1937); The Egyptian names are only given where there is some degree of certainty about the identification.

Cabbage (*Brassica oleracea*)	Fennel (*Foeniculum vulgare*)	Mint (*Mentha sativa*)	Radish (*Raphanus sativus*)
Calamus (*Acorus calamus*)	Fenugreek (*Trigonella foenum-graecum*)	Moringa (*Moringa pterygosperma*) (Egyptian: *b3ḳ*)	Ricinus (*Ricinus communis*)(Egyptian: *dgm*)
Caraway (*Carum carvi*)	Fir (*Abies cilicica*)	Mustard (*Sinapis alba*)	Saffron (*Saffron crocus*)
Carob (*Ceratonia siliqua*)	Flax (*Linum usitatissimum*)	Myrrh (*Commiphora Molmol*)	Sebesten

Parts of plants

Bean (*Vigna sinensis*)	Blossom	Fruit	Resin	Thorn
Berry	Fig (*Ficus carica*)(Egyptian: *d3b*)	Nut	Seed	

Products from plants

Beer (Egyptian: *ḥnḳt*)	Dough	Gum	Sawdust
Bran	Flour	Juice	Tar
Bread	Frankincense	Oil	Wine (Egyptian: *irp*)

Animal kingdom

Names of animals

Ass	Dog	Hippopotamus	Mole	Scorpion
Bat	Duck	Ibex	Mouse	Sheep
Bee	Eel	Ibis	Pelican	Swallow
Beetle	Fly	Lion	Ostrich	Swordfish
Cat	Frog	Lizard	Ox	Tadpole
Cow	Gazelle	Locust	Pelican	Tortoise
Crab	Goat	Man	Pig	Vulture
Crocodile	Goose	Millipede	Ram	Worm

Parts of animals

Bile	Feather	Leg	Slough	Viscera
Blood	Flesh	Liver	Spine	Vulva
Bone	Hair	Marrow	Spleen	Womb
Brain	Head	Phallus	Tail	
Dung	Hoof	Semen	Teeth	
Ear	Horn	Shell	Testicle	
Eye	Fluid	Skull	Urine	

Products of animals

Egg	Fat	Honey (Egyptian: *bit*)	Milk (Egyptian: *irtt*)	Wax

Mineral kingdom

Names of minerals

Alabaster	Chalcedony	Hematite	Mud	Salt (Egyptian: *ḥm3t*)
Alum	Chalcopyrite	Lapis lazuli	Naphtha	Soot
Antimony	Chrysocoll	Lead	Natron (Egyptian: *ḥsmn*)	Stibium
Arsenic sulphide	Copper	Limestone	Ochre	
Asphalt	Faience	Magnetite	Orpiment	
Bitumen	Granite	Malachite	Pumice stone	
Calamine	Gypsum	Millstone scraping	Rust	

Products from minerals

Brick	Clay	Dye	Eye-paint	Ink-powder

Bibliography

Adams, Michael P. *et al.* (2005). *Pharmacology for Nurses: A Pathophysiologic Approach*. Prentice Hall: Upper Saddle River, N.J.

Ang-Lee, M. K. (2002). 'Most commonly used herbal medicines in the USA' *Textbook of Complementary and Alternative Medicine*. ed. Chun-Su Yuan. Parthenon Pub. Group: Boca Raton.

Assmann, Jan (1990). *Ma'at: Gerechtigkeit und Unsterblichkeit im Alten Ägypten*. Beck: München.

Badr, MM. (1963). 'The history of urology in ancient Egypt' *Journal of the International College of Surgeons* 39: 404–13.

Banov, Leon Jr. (1965). 'The Chester Beatty medical papyrus: The earliest known treatise completely devoted to anorectal diseases' *Surgery* 58: 1037–43.

Banu, Ion (1967). "Le papyrus medical Edwin Smith, considere au point de vue philosophique" *Studia et Acta Orientalia* 5–6: 117–41.

Bardinet, Thierry (1995). *Les Papyrus Médicaux de l'Égypte Pharaonique*. Fayard: Paris.

——— (1999). 'La mouche et l'abeille: l'utilisation de la propolis d'après les textes médicaux de l'Égypte pharaonique, deuxième partie; Les emplois thérapeutiques' *Göttinger Miszellen* 171: 23–41.

Bardis, P. (1967). 'Circumcision in ancient Egypt' *Indian Journal of the History of Medicine* 12(1): 22–3.

——— (1968). 'Contraception in ancient Egypt' *Indian Journal of the History of Medicine* 12(2): 305–7.

Barker, Ernest (1946). *The Politics of Aristotle*. Clarendon Press: Oxford.

Basham, A. L. (1976). 'The practice of medicine in ancient and medieval India' ed. Charles Lesile *Asian Medical Systems: A Comparative Study*. University of California Press: Berkeley. 18–43.

Bennett, Richard N. *et al.* (1994). 'Tansley review No. 72. Secondary metabolites in plant defence mechanisms' *New Phytologist* 127: 617–33.

Bergman, A. *et al.* (1983). 'Acceleration of wound healing by topical application of honey' *The American Journal of Surgery* 145: 374–5.

Betz, H. D. (1986). *The Greek Magical Papyri in Translation*. The University of Chicago Press: Chicago.

Biggs, Robert D. (1995). 'Medicine, surgery, and public health in ancient Mesopotamia' *Civilizations of the Ancient Near East*, vol. 3: Scribner: New York. 1911–24.

Bisset, Norman G. *et al.* (1994). 'Was opium known in 18th dynasty ancient Egypt? An examination of materials from the tomb of the chief royal architect Kha' *Journal of Ethnopharmacology* 41: 99–114.

——— (1996). 'The presence of opium in a 3,500 Year Old Cypriote Base-Ring juglet' *Ägypten und Levante* 6: 203–4.

Blackman, Winifred S. (2000). *The Felläḥīn of Upper Egypt: With a New Forword by Salima Ikram*. The American University in Cairo Press: Cairo (originally published in 1927, London).

Breasted, J. H. (1930). *The Edwin Smith Papyrus*. The University of Chicago Press: Chicago.

Bryant, Bronwen Jean *et al.* (2003). *Pharmacology for Health Professionals*. Mosby/Elsevier Science: Marrickville.

Budge, W. (1928). *The Divine Origin of the Craft of the Herbalist*. Dover Publications: New York.

Burger, Alfred (1995). *Understanding Medications: What the Label doesn't Tell You*. American Chemical Society: Washington, DC.

Burkert, Walter (1972). *Lore and science in ancient Pythagoreanism*. trans. Edwin L. Minar, Jr. Harvard University Press: Cambridge, Mass.

Cave, A. J. E. (1950). 'Ancient Egypt and the origin of anatomical science' *Proceedings of the Royal Society of Medicine* 43: 568–71.

Chace, Arnold Buffum (1929). *The Rhind Mathematical Papyrus*. National Council of Teachers of Mathematics: Reston.

Chadwick, J. *et al.* (1978). *Hippocratic Writings*. ed. Lloyd G. E. R. Penguin Books: New York.

Chassinate, E. G. (1921). 'Un papyrus medical Copte' *Mémoires Publiés par les Membres de l'Institut Français d'Archéologie Orientale du Caire*, vol. 32.

Chevallier, Andrew (1996). *The Encyclopedia of Medicinal Plants*. DK Adult: New York.

——— (2000). *Encyclopedia of Herbal Medicine*. DK Adult: New York.

Clark, David E. *et al.* (2000) 'Computational methods for the prediction of "drug-likeness" ' *Drug Discovery Today* 5: 49–58.

Clendening, Logan (1960). *Source Book of Medical History*. Dover Publications: New York.

Cole, Dorothea (1986). 'Obstetrics for the women of ancient Egypt' *Discussions in Egyptology* 5: 27–33.

Comrie, John D. (1909). 'Medicine among the Assyrians and Egyptians in 1500 BC' *Edinburgh Medical Journal* 2: 101–29.

Dawson, Warren Royal (1923–24). 'Egyptian medicine under the Copts in the early Centuries of Christian era' *Proceedings of the Royal Society of Medicine* 17: 51–7.

——— (1924). 'The mouse in Egyptian and later medicine' *Proceedings of the Royal Society of Medicine* 10: 83–6.

——— (1925). 'Bats as materia medica' *Annals and Magazine of Natural History* 16: 221–7.

——— (1927). 'Early ideas relating to conception, contraconception, and sex-determination' *The Caledonian Medical Journal* 13: 296–302.

——— (1929). 'Studies in medical history (a) The origin of herbal (b) Castor-oil in Antiquity' *Aegyptus* 10: 47–72.

——— (1932a). 'A strange drug' *Aegyptus* 12: 12–16.

——— (1932b). 'Studies in the Egyptian medical texts' *Journal of Egyptian Archaeology* 18: 150–4.

——— (1932–33). 'The earliest surgical treatise' *The British Journal of Surgery* 20: 34–43.

——— (1933). 'Studies in the Egyptian medical texts' *Journal of Egyptian Archaeology* 19: 133–7.

——— (1934). 'Studies in the Egyptian medical texts' *Journal of Egyptian Archaeology* 20: 41–6, 185–8.

——— (1935). 'Studies in the Egyptian medical texts' *Journal of Egyptian Archaeology* 21: 37–40.

——— (1964). *Beginnings: Egypt & Assyria.* Hafner Publishing Company: New York.

Dunand, Françoise *et al.* (2004). *Gods and Men in Egypt 3000 BCE to 395 CE.* trans. David Lorton. Cornell University Press: Ithaca, London.

Ebadi, Manuchair (2002). *Pharmacodynamic Basis of Herbal Medicine.* CRC: Boca Raton, London.

Ebbell, B. (1928). 'Die ägyptischen Krankheitsnamen' *Zeitschrift für ägyptische Sprache und Altertumskunde* 63: 71–5, 115–21.

——— (1937). *The Papyrus Ebers.* Oxford University Press: London.

Ebers, G. M. (1875). *Papyros Ebers* (two volumes). Englemann: Leipzig.

Edel, Elmar (1976). *Ägyptische Ärzte und ägyptische Medizin am hethitischen Königshof: neue Funde von Keilschriftbriefen Ramses' II. aus Boğazköy.* Westdeutscher Verlag: Opladen.

Edelstein, Ludwig (1970). 'Galen' *The Oxford Classical Dictionary.* ed. Hammond N. G. L. *et al.* Clarendon Press: Oxford. 454–5.

Edghill, E. A. *et al.* (1963). 'Pentateuch' ed. Frederick C. Grant and H. H. Rowley *Dictionary of the Bible.* Scribner: New York. 744–8.

Erman, Adolf (1894, reprinted in 1969). *Life in Ancient Egypt.* trans. H. M. Tirard. B. Blom: New York.

Erman, Adolf *et al.* (1925–55). *Wörterbuch der Ägyptischen Sprache* vol. 1–5. Akadamie-Verlag: Berlin.

Estes, J Worth (1993). *The Medical Skills of Ancient Egypt.* Science History Publications: Canton.

Faulkner, R. O. (1962). *A Concise Dictionary of Middle Egyptian.* University Press: Oxford.

——— (1972). *The Ancient Egyptian Book of the Dead.* British Museum Publications: London.

Foster, John L. (2001). *Ancient Egyptian Literature: An Anthology.* University of Texas Press: Austin.

Frankfort, Henri (1961). *Ancient Egyptian Religion: An Interpretation.* Harper: New York.

Fraser, Peter Marshall (1972). *Ptolemaic Alexandria.* Clarendon Press: Oxford.

Froehner, R. (1934). 'Der Veterinärpapyrus von Kahun' *Deutsche tierärztliche Wochenschrift* 42: 704–9.

el-Gammal, Samir Yahia (1989). 'Egyptian pharmacy in Chassinet Coptic Papyrus' *Proceeding of the XIXth International Congress of Papyrology* 1: 723–35.

Gardiner, A. H. (1915). 'Magic' *Encyclopaedia of Religion and Ethics* 8: 262–9.

——— (1938). 'The house of life" *Journal of Egyptian Archaeology* 24: 157–79.

——— (1957). *Egyptian Grammar.* 3rd ed. Oxford University: London.

Germer, Renate (1979). *Untersuchung über Arzneimittelpflanzen im Alten Ägypten.* Dissertation: Hamburg.

——— (1980). 'Lattich' *Lexikon der Ägyptologie* vol. 3. ed. Wolfgang Helck and Eberhard Otto. O. Harrassowitz: Wiesbaden. 938–9.

——— (1993). 'Ancient Egyptian pharmaceutical plants' *The Healing Past: Pharmaceutical in the Biblical and Rabbinic World.* ed. Walter Jacob *et al.* E.J. Brill: Leiden.

——— (2002). *Die Heilpflanzen der Ägypter.* Artemis & Winkler: Düsseldorf.

Ghalioungui, Paul (1960). 'Dès papyrus Égyptiens a la médecine Grecque' *XVIIe Congrès international d'histoire de la médecine.* 296–306.

——— (1961). 'Medicine under the ancient Egyptians' *Egyptian Travel Magazine* 77: 16–20.

——— (1966a). 'The spiral course of medical thinking' *Journal of Egypt Public Health Association* 41: 127–31.

——— (1967a). 'La notion de maladie dans les textes Égyptiens et ses rapports avex la théorie humorale' *Bulletin de l'Institut Français d'Archéologie Orientale* 65: 37–48.

——— (1967b). 'Quelques apercus de la Médecine Pharaonique' *Revue Medicale de la Suisser Romande* 87: 837–52.

——— (1968). 'The relation of Pharaonic to Greek and later medicine' *Bulletin of the Cleveland Medical Library* 15: 96–107.

——— (1969a). 'Ancient Egyptian remedies and Mediaeval Arabic writers' *Bulletin de l'Institut Français d'Archéologie Orientale* 68: 41–6.

——— (1969b). 'La medecine pharaonique ses origines, ses realisations, son heritage' *Le Journal Medical Libanais* 22: 159–70.

——— (1971). 'Did a dental profession exist in Ancient Egypt?' *Medical History* 15: 92–4.

——— (1973). *Magic and Medical Science in Ancient Egypt.* 2nd ed. B. M. Israël: Amsterdam.

——— (1977). 'The persistence and spread of some obstetric concepts held in ancient Egypt' *Annales du Service des Antiquités de l'Egypte* 62: 141–5.

——— (1983). *The Physicians of Pharaonic Egypt*. Al-Ahram Center for Scientific Translations: Cairo.

——— (1984). 'Four landmarks of Egyptian cardiology' *Journal of the Royal College of Physicians of London* 18: 182–6.

——— (1986). 'A comparison between the medical plant mentioned in Greco-Roman and ancient Egyptian papyri' *Bulletin of the Center of Papyrological Studies* 3: 9–16.

——— (1987). *The Ebers Papyrus*. Academy of Scientific Research and Technology: Cairo.

Ghalioungui, Paul *et al.* (1963). 'On an ancient Egyptian method of diagnosing pregnancy and determining foetal sex' *Medical Historian* 7: 241–3.

Ghalioungui, Paul and Guindi, S. (1966b). 'The persistence of the use of catamenial and uterine blood in folk medicine' *Bulletin de l'Institut Égyptien* 47: 65–8.

Gordon, Andrew H. and Schwabe, Calvin W. (2004). *The Quick and the Dead: Biomedical Theory in Ancient Egypt*. Brill-Styx: Boston.

Grapow, H., von Deines, H. and Westendorf, W. (1954–73). *Grundriß der Medizin der Alten Ägypter* (9 volumes). Akademie-Verlag: Berlin.

Green, Lyn (2003). 'Beyond the humors: Some thoughts on comparisons between Pharaonic and Greco-Roman medicine' *Egyptology at the Dawn of the Twenty-first Century*, vol.2. American University in Cairo Press: Cairo.

Griffith, F. L. (1891). 'The metrology of the medical papyrus Ebers' *Proceedings of the Society of Biblical Archaeology* 13: 392–406, 526–38.

Griffiths, John G. (1982). 'Osiris' *Lexikon der Ägyptologie* vol. 4. ed. Wolfgang Helck and Eberhard Otto. O. Harrassowitz: Wiesbaden. 623–33.

Guili, Zheng (1997). *Concise Chinese Materia Medica*. trans. Yang Huiqin. Shandong Science and Technology Press: Jinan.

Gundlach, Rolf (1986). 'Vergangenheit, Verhältnis zur' *Lexikon der Ägyptologie* vol. 6. ed. Wolfgang Helck and Eberhard Otto. O. Harrassowitz: Wiesbaden. 981–5.

Habachi, Labib and Ghalipongui, Paul (1969–70). 'Note on nine physicians of pharaonic Egypt of whom five hitherto unknown' *Bulletin de l'Institut Égyptien* 51: 15–23.

Halioua, Bruno *et al.* (2005). *Medicine in the Days of the Pharaohs*. Belknap Press of Harvard University Press: Cambridge, MA.

Harris, J. R. (1971). *The Legacy of Egypt*. Clarendon Press: Oxford.

Hart, George (1986). *A Dictionary of Egyptian Gods and Goddesses*. Routledge & Kegan Paul: London, Boston.

Hongtu, Wang (1999). *Clinical Applications: The Yellow Emperor's Canon on Internal Medicine*. trans. Li Yachan. New World Press: Beijing.

Horgan, E. S. (1949). 'Medicine and surgery in the most ancient East: Babylonia and Egypt' *Sudan Notes & Records* 30: 29–46.

Houten, T. (1980). 'The Edwin Smith papyrus 1: The surgical management of cranial injuries' *Museum Applied Science Center for Archaeology Journal* 1: 99–101.

Howe, David (2001). *Data Analysis for Database Design*. 3rd ed. Butterworth-Heinemann: Oxford.

Hussein, Mahmoud I. (1998). 'The medical title *wr swnw pr-ˁ3 ḫrp msḥm 3ˁˁ mw m-ẖnw nṯnṯ.t*' *Discussion in Egyptology* 42: 55–68.

——— (2001). 'The medical title *swnw pr-ˁ3 ˁw hmwt st3t*' *Discussion in Egyptology* 50: 25–31.

Iversen, Erik (1953). 'Wounds in the head in Egyptian and Hippocratic medicine' *Studia Orientalia Ioanni Pedersen*. Einar Munksgaard: Copenhagen. 163–71.

Jacob, Irene. (1993). 'Ricinus Communis: The miracle tree through four thousand years' *The Healing Past: Pharmaceutical in the Biblical and Rabbinic World*. ed. Walter Jacob *et al.* E. J. Brill: Leiden. 81–93.

Jacob, Walter (1993). 'Medicinal plants of the bible: Another view' *The Healing Past: Pharmaceutical in the Biblical and Rabbinic World*. ed. Walter Jacob *et al.* E. J. Brill: Leiden. 27–46.

Jagtap, A. G. *et al.* (2004). 'Effect of polyherbal formulation on experimental models of inflammatory bowel diseases' *Journal of Ethnopharmacology* 90: 195–204.

Jonckheere, Frans (1944). *Une maladie égyptienne, l'hématurie parasitaire*. Fondation Égyptologique Reine Élizabeth: Brussels.

——— (1951). 'Le cadre professionnel et administratif des médecins égyptiens' *Chronique d'Egypte* 26: 237–68.

——— (1958). *Les Médecins de l'Égypte Pharaonique: Essai de Prosopographie*. Fondation Égyptologique Reine Élisabeth Parc du Cinquantenaire: Bruxelles.

Jones, W. H. S. (1931). *Hippocrates: With an English Translation by W. H. S. Jones* vol. 4. William Heinemann LTD: London.

Jouanna, J. (2004). 'Médecine égyptienne et médecine grecque' *La Médecine grecque antique: Actes du 14e Colloque de la Villa Kérylos à Beaulieu-sur-mer*. 15: 1-21.

Kachigan, Sam Kash (1991). *Multivariate Statistical Analysis: A Conceptual Introduction*. Radius Press: New York.

Karenberg, A. and Christian Leitz. (2001) 'Headache in magical and medical papyri of ancient Egypt' *Cephalalgia* 21: 911–16.

Kenner, Dan (1996). *Botanical Medicine*. Paradigm Publications: Brookline, Mass.

Keswani, N. H. (1967). 'Ancient Hindu orthopaedic surgery' *Indian Journal of Orthopaedics* 1: 76–94.

King, Helen (2001). *Greek and Roman Medicine*. Bristol Classical Press: London.

King, S. Lester (1982). *Medical Thinking: A Historical Preface*. Princeton University Press: Princeton.

von Klein, Carl H. (1905). 'The medical features of the papyrus Ebers' *The Journal of the American Medical Association* 45: 1928–35.

Kolta, Kamal Sabri *et al.* (2000). ' "Schmerzen", "Schmerzstoffe" oder "Fäulnisprinzip"? Zur Bedeutung von *wḫdw*, einem zentralen Terminus der altägyptischen Medizin' *Zeitschrift für ägyptische Sprache und Altertumskunde* 127: 38–52.

Koschel, Klaus (1996). 'Opium Alkaloids in a Cypriote Base Ring I Vessel (Bilbil) of the Middle Bronze Age from Egypt' *Ägypten und Levante* 6: 159–66.

Krikorian, A. D. (1978). 'Were the Opium Poppy and Opium Known in the Ancient Near East?' *Journal of the History of Biology* 8: 94–114.

Kutumbiah, P. (1957). 'Tubular system of the body. Ancient Egyptian and Hindu medical views' *Indian Journal of the History of Medicine* 2: 13–20.

Leake, Chauncey Depew (1940). 'Ancient Egyptian therapeutics' *Ciba Symposia* 1: 311–22.

——— (1952). *The Old Egyptian Medical Papyri.* University of Kansas Press: Kansas.

Leek, F. Filce. (1969). 'Did a dental profession exist in ancient Egypt?' *The Dental Delineator* 20: 18–21.

——— (1972). 'Did a dental profession exist in ancient Egypt during the 3rd Millennium B.C.?' *Medical History* 16: 404–6.

Lefebvre, G. (1952). 'Tableau des parties du corps humain mentionnées par les Égptiens' *Supplément aux Annales du Service des Antiquités, IFAO* 17.

——— (1956). *Essai sur la médecine égyptienne de l'époque pharaonique.* Presses Universitaires de France: Paris.

Leitz, Christian (1999). *Magical and Medical Papyri of the New Kingdom.* British Museum Press for the Trustees of the British Museum: London.

——— (2005). 'Die Rolle von Religion und Naturbeobachtung bei der Auswahl der Drogen im Papyrus Ebers' *Papyrus Ebers und die antike Heilkunde: Akten der Tagung vom 15.-16. 3. 2002 in der Albertina/ UB der Universität Leipzig.* Harrassowitz: Wiesbaden. 41–62.

Le Roux, Brigitte *et al.* (2004). *Geometric Data Analysis: From Correspondence Analysis to Structured Data Analysis.* Kluwer Academic Publishers: Dordrecht, Boston.

Lesile, Charles (1976). *Asian medical systems: a comparative study.* University of California Press: Berkeley.

Lichtheim, Miriam (1973). *Ancient Egyptian Literature: A Book of Readings* vol. 1. University of California Press: Berkeley.

——— (1976). *Ancient Egyptian Literature: A Book of Readings* vol. 2. University of California Press: Berkeley.

Long, Bernard. (1984). 'A propos de l'usage des menthes dans l'Egypte ancienne' *Mélanges Adolphe Gutbub* 1: 145–59.

Longrigg, James (1998). *Greek Medicine from the Heroic to the Hellenistic Age: A Source Book.* Routledge: New York.

Macaulay, G. C. (1904). *The History of Herodotus*, vol. 1. The Macmillan Company: New York.

Majno, Guido M. D. (1975). *The Healing Hand.* Harvard University Press: Cambridge, Mass.

Manly, Bryan F. J. (1994). Multivariate StatisticalMethods: A Primer. 2nd ed. Chapman & Hall: London.

Mann, John (2000). *Murder, Magic, and Medicine.* Oxford University Press: New York.

Manniche, L. (1989). *An Ancient Egyptian Herbal.* British Museum Press: London.

——— (1999). *Sacred Luxuries: Fragrance, Aromatherapy and Cosmetics in Ancient Egypt.* Opus Publishing Limited: London.

Marganne, Marie-Helene. (1993). 'Links between Egypt and Greek medicine' *Experimental and Clinical Medicine* 3: 35–43.

Maspéro, Gaston. (1909). *New light on ancient Egypt.* trans. Elizabeth Lee. T.F. Unwin: London.

Merrillees, R. S. (1962). 'Opium trade in the Bronze Age Levant' *Antiquity* 36: 287–92.

Merskey, H. (1989). 'The womb lay still in ancient Egypt' *British Journal of Psychiatry* 154: 751–3.

Meulnaere, Herman J. (1975). 'Ärzteschule' *Lexikon der Ägyptologie* vol. 1. ed. Wolfgang Helck and Eberhard Otto. O. Harrassowitz: Wiesbaden. 80.

Meulenbeld, Jan G. (1987). 'Reflections on the basic concepts of Indian pharmacology' ed. Jan Meulenbeld *Studies on Indian Medical History.* Egbert Forsten: Groningen.

Meyerhof, Max (1940). 'Eye disease in ancient Egypt' *Ciba Symposia* 1: 305–10.

Miller, Robert (1994). '*Ḏaajs*, Peganum Harmala L' *Bulletin de l'Institut Français d'Archéologie Orientale* 94: 349–57.

Nunn, John F. (1996). *Ancient Egyptian Medicine.* British Museum Press: London.

Obeyesekere, Gananath (1976). 'The impact of Āyurvedic ideas on the culture and the individual in Sri Lanka' ed. Charles Lesile *Asian Medical Systems: A Comparative Study.* University of California Press: Berkeley. 201–26.

Ockinga, Boyo (1983). 'The burden of KHAʿKH EPERRĒʿSONBU' *Journal of Egyptian Archaeology* 69: 88–95.

——— (2001). 'Ethics and morality' *The Oxford encyclopedia of ancient Egypt.* ed Donald B. Redford. Oxford University Press: New York. 484–7.

von Oefele, Felix Freiherr (1908). 'Zur Quellenscheidung des Papyrus Ebers' *Archiv für Geschichte der Medizin* 1: 12–28, 122–40.

Oldfather, C. H. (1933). *Diodorus of Sicily with an English Translation*, vol. 1. William Heinemann Ltd.: London.

Otsuka, Yasuo (1976). 'Chinese traditional medicine in Japan' ed. Charles Lesile *Asian Medical Systems: A Comparative Study.* University of California Press: Berkeley. 322–40.

Pahor, Ahms L. (1992). 'Ear, nose and throat in ancient Egypt' *The Journal of Laryngology and Otology* 106: 677–87, 773–9, 863–73.

——— (2003). 'Pharaonic ORL' *International Congress Series* 1240: 1349–59.

Parker, Richard A. (1952). 'Sothic dates and calendar "adjustment" ' *Revue d'Egyptologie* 9: 101–8.

Philip, J. A. (1966). *Pythagoras and Early Pythagoreanism.* University of Toronto Press: Toronto.

Pinch, G. (1994). *Magic in Ancient Egypt.* British Museum Press: London.

Pommerening, Tanja (2003). 'Altägyptische Rezepturen metrologisch neu interpretiert' *Berichte zur Wissenschaftsgeschichte* 26: 1–16.

Poole, Federico (2001). 'Cumin set milk, honey: An ancient Egyptian medicine container' *Journal of Egyptian Archaeology* 87: 175–80.

Porter, Roy (1997). *The Greatest Benefit to Mankind.* Harper Collins: London.

Potter, Paul (1995). *Hippocrates*, vol. 8. Harvard University Press: Cambridge.

Prioreschi, Plinio (1993). 'Skull trauma in Egyptian and Hippocratic medicine' *Gesnerus* 50: 167–78.

——— (2003). 'Egyptian and Greek medicine' *Turkish Journal of Medical Ethics, Law, and History* 11: 149–61.

Qingye, Li (1998). *Formulas of Traditional Chinese Medicine.* Xue yuan chu ban she: Beijing.

Quack, Joachim Friedrich (1999) 'Ein neues medizinisches Fragment der Spätzeit (pAshmolean Museum 1984.55 rt.)' *Zeitschrift für ägyptische Sprache und Altertumskunde* 126: 141–49.

——— (2003). 'Methoden und Möglichkeiten der Erforschung der Medizin im Alten Ägypten' *Medizinhistorisches Journal* 38: 3–15.

Ramachandra, Rao S. K. (ed) (1985). *Encyclopaedia of Indian Medicine*, vol. 1. Kalpatharu Res. Acad: Bangalore.

Ranke, Hermann (1941). 'Medicine and Surgery in Ancient Egypt' *University of Pennsylvania Bicentennial Conference: Studies in the History of Science.* Pennsylvania University Press: Philadelphia.

Raskin, Iiya *et al.* (2002). 'Plants and human health in the twenty-first century' *Trends in Biotechnology* 20: 522–9.

Reeves, C. (1980). 'Illustration of medicine in Ancient Egypt' *The Journal of audiovisual media in medicine* 3: 4–13.

——— (1992). *Egyptian Medicine.* Shire Publications Ltd.: London.

Reymond, Eve Anne E. (1976). *A Medical Book from Crocodilopolis.* Verlag Brüder Hollinek: Vienna.

——— (1984). 'From an ancient Egyptian dentist's handbook P.Vindob. D. 12287' *Melanges Adolphe Gutbub.* Université de Montpellier: Montpellier. 183–99.

Richard J. Ablin (1996) 'AIDS: Déjà Vu in Ancient Egypt?' *Emerging Infectious Diseases*, vol. 2, no. 3. URL: http://www.cdc.gov/ncidod/eid/vol2no3/letters.htm.

Richardson, M. E. J. (2004). *Hammurabi's Law: Text, Translation and Glossary.* T&T Clark International: London, New York.

Ritner, Robert K. (1989). 'Horus on the Crocodiles: A juncture of religion and magic in Late Dynastic Egypt.' ed. Simpson W. K. *Religion and Philosophy in Ancient Egypt.* Yale Egyptological Seminar: New Haven, Conneticut. 103–16.

——— (2000). 'Innovations and adaptations in ancient Egyptian medicine' *Journal of Near Eastern Studies* 59: 107–17.

——— (2001a). 'Magic' *The Oxford Encyclopedia of Ancient Egypt*, vol. 2. ed. Donald B. Redford. Oxford University Press: New York. 321–36.

——— (2001b). 'Medicine' *The Oxford Encyclopedia of Ancient Egypt*, vol. 2. ed. Donald B. Redford. Oxford University Press: New York. 353–6.

Rhodes, Philip (1985). *An Outline History of Medicine.* Butterworths: London, Boston.

Ruffer, M. A. (1921). *Studies in Palaeopathology of Egypt.* ed. R. L. Moodie. University of Chicago Press: Chicago.

Saunders, J B de CM. (1963). *The Transitions from Ancient Egypt to Greek Medicine.* University of Kansas Press: Lawrence.

Säve-Söderbergh, T. (1961). *Pharaohs and Mortals.* trans. R. E. Oldenburg. Bobbs-Merrill: Indianapolis.

Schwabe, C. W. (1986). 'Bull semen and muscle ATP: Some evidence of the dawn of medical science in ancient Egypt' *Canadian Journal of Veterinary Research* 50: 145–53.

Sélincourt, A. D. (1996). *Herodotus: The Histories.* Penguin Books: London, New York.

Shelton, W. Jay. (2004). *Homeopathy : how it really works.* Prometheus Books: Amherst.

Siegel, Andrew F. (1996). Statistics and data analysis : an introduction. J. Wiley: New York.

Sigerist, Henry E. (1951). *A History of Medicine*, vol. 1. Oxford University Press: New York.

Silver, E. H. and Kemper K. J. (1999). *White Willow Bark (Salix alba).* URL: http://www.longwoodherbal.org/willowbark/willow.pdf.

Sims, Randi L. (1999). *Bivariate Data Analysis : A Practical Guide.* Nova Science: New York.

Sivin, Nathan (1995). *Medicine, Philosophy and Religion in Ancient China: Researches and Reflection.* Ashgate Publishing Ltd.: Aldershot.

Skeat, Walter William (1901). *A Concise Etymological Dictionary of the English Language.* Clarendon Press: Oxford.

Sobhy, George P. G. (1938). 'Remains of ancient Egyptian medicine in modern domestic treatment' *Bulletin de l'Institut Égyptien* 20: 9–18.

——— (1950). 'The persistence of ancient Coptic methods of medical treatment in present-day Egypt' *Coptic Studies in Honor of Walter Ewing Crum.* Boston, Mass: 185–8.

——— (1952). 'Studies in ancient Egyptian medicine: Comparison of the medical treatment of intestinal worms in ancient Egypt with the present day folklore and domestic medicines in Egypt' *Archiv Orientální. Journal of the Czechoslovak Oriental Institute* 20: 626–8.

von Staden, Heinrich (1989). *Herophilus: The Art of Medicine in Early Alexandria*. Cambridge University Press: Cambridge.

——— (1992). 'Affinities and elisions: Helen and Hellenocentrism' *Isis* 83: 578–95.

Steiner, Richard (1992). 'Northwest Semetic Incantations in ancient Egyptian Medical Papyrus of the Fourteenth Century B.C.E.' *Journal of Near Eastern Studies* 51: 191–200.

Stephan, Joachim (1997). 'Überlegungen zur Ausbildung der Ärzte im alten Ägypten' *Studien zur Altägyptischen Kultur* 24: 301–23.

——— (2001). *Ordnungssysteme in der altäyptischen Medizin und ihre Überlieferung in den europäischen Kulturkreis*. PhD thesis: Universität Hamburg.

——— (2005). 'Medizinschulen im Alten Ägypten und der Einfluß ihrer Lehren auf die griechische Medizin'' *Papyrus Ebers und die antike Heilkunde: Akten der Tagung vom 15.-16. 3. 2002 in der Albertina/UB der Universität Leipzig*. Harrassowitz: Wiesbaden. 81–101.

Stetter, C. (1993). *The Secret Medicine of the Pharaohs*. Edition q: Chicago.

Steuer, Robert O. (1948). '*wḫdw*: aetiological principle of pyaemia in ancient Egyptian medicine' *Bulletin of History of Medicine*. Supplement 10.

——— (1961). 'Controversial problems concerning the interpretation of the Physiological treatises of Papyrus Ebers' *Isis* 52: 372–80.

Steuer, Robert O. and Saunders, J B de CM. (1959). *Ancient Egyptian & Cnidian Medicine*. University of California Press: Berkeley, Los Angeles.

Stevens, J. M. (1975). 'Gynaeocology from ancient Egypt; The Papyrus Kahun' *Medical Journal of Australia* 2: 949–52.

Tait, W. J. (1991). 'P. Carlsberg 230: Eleven fragments from a demotic herbal' *The Carlsberg Papyri 1: Demotic Texts from the Collection*. ed. Frandsen Carstan P. J. Niebuhr Institute Publications: Copenhagen. 47–92.

Tapp, E. (1979). 'Diseases in the Manchester mummies' *Science in Egyptology*. ed. David, A. R. Manchester University Press: Manchester.

Teeter, Emily (2001). 'Maat' *The Oxford Encyclopedia of Ancient Egypt*, vol. 2. ed. Redford, Donald B. Oxford University Press: New York. 319–21.

Temkin, Owsei (1938). 'The papyrus Ebers' *Isis* 28: 126–31.

Temkin, Owsei *et al.* (1967). *Ancient Medicine*. The Johns Hopkins Press: Baltimore.

Thissen, Heinz-Josef (1977). 'Hermetische Schriften' *Lexikon der Ägyptologie* vol. 2. ed. Wolfgang Helck and Eberhard Otto. O. Harrassowitz: Wiesbaden. 1135–7.

Thorwald, Jürgen (1962). *Science and Secrets of Early Medicine: Egypt, Mesopotamia, India, China, Mexico, Peru*. trans. Richard and Clara Winston. Thames & Hudson: London.

Unschuld, Paul Ulrich (1985). *Medicine in China: a history of ideas*. University of California Press: Berkeley.

Waddell, W. G. (1940). *Manetho: With an English Translation by W.G. Waddell*. Harvard University Press: Cambridge, Mass.

Wagner, H. (2000). 'New targets in phytopharmacology of plants' *Herbal Medicine: A Concise Overview for Professionals*. ed. Edzard, H. Butterworth-Heinemann: Boston.

Walker, H. James (1990). 'The place of magic in the practice of medicine in ancient Egypt' *The Bulletin of the Australian Centre for Egyptology* 1: 85–95.

——— (1996). *Studies in Ancient Egyptian Anatomical Terminology*. Aris and Phillips: Warminster.

Walker, John (1934). *Folk Medicine in Modern Egypt*. Luzac: London.

Walker, R. E. (1964). 'The veterinary papyrus of Kahun' *The Veterinary Record* 76: 198–200.

Warrier, Gopi *et al.* (1997). *The Complete Illustrated Guide to Ayurveda: The Ancient Indian Healing Tradition*. Element: Rockport, Mass.

Weber, M. (1980). 'Lebenshaus' *Lexikon der Ägyptologie* vol. 3. ed. Wolfgang Helck and Eberhard Otto. O. Harrassowitz: Wiesbaden. 954–8.

Wiseman, Nigel (1995). *Fundamentals of Chinese medicine*. Paradigm Publications: Brookline, Mass.

Weeks, Kent R. (1976–78). 'Studies of Papyrus Ebers' *Bulletin de l'Institut d'Egypte* 58–9: 292–9.

——— (1980). 'Ancient Egyptian dentistry' *An X-Ray Atlas of the Royal Mummies*. ed. James Harris. University of Chicago Press: Chicago.

——— (1995). 'Medicine, surgery and public health in ancient Egypt' *Civilization of the Ancient Near East*, vol. 3. Charles Scribner's Sons: New York.

Weinberger, Bernhard Wolf (1932). 'The practice of Egyptian dentistry as revealed in the Edwin Smith surgical papyrus' *8e Congrès Dentaire International* 16: 56–62.

Weser, Ulrich (1987). "Biochemical Basis of Copper in Ancient Egyptian and Roman Medicine" ed. James Black *Recent Advances in the Conservation and Analysis of Artifacts*. Summer Schools Press: London. 189–93.

Westendorf, Wolfhart (1992). *Erwachen der Heilkunst: Die Medizin in Alten Ägypten*. Artemis & Winkler: Zürich.

——— (1999). *Handbuch der Altägyptischen Medizin*. Brill: Leiden, Boston.

Williamson, E. M. (2000). 'Synergy—myth or reality?' ed. Edzard Ernst. *Herbal Medicine: A Concise Overview for Professionals*. Butterworth-Heinemann: Boston. 41–58.

Wreszinski, W. (1913). *Der Papyrus Ebers: Umschrift, Übersetzung und Kommentar*. Hinrichs: Leipzig.

Xingdong, He (1998). *The Chinese Materia Medica.* Xue yuan chu ban she: Beijing.
Yahuda, A. S. (1947). 'Medical and anatomical terms in the Pentateuch in the light of Egyptian medical papyri' *Journal of the History of Medicine and Allied Sciences* 2: 549–74.
Yanchi, Liu (1998). *Basic theories of traditional Chinese medicine.* Xue yuan chu ban she: Beijing.

General Index

Index of Citations of Medical Papyri

Ebers Papyrus

Eb.422	54
Eb.437	36
Eb.467	38
Eb.468	54
Eb.469	24
Eb.474	37
Eb.482	37
Eb.491	39
Eb.499	28, 55
Eb.500	28, 55
Eb.509	56
Eb.511	28
Eb.522	3
Eb.533	39
Eb.565	42
Eb.580	40
Eb.582	65
Eb.587	3
Eb.594	42
Eb.605	3
Eb.609	3
Eb.617	26
Eb.630	3
Eb.636	56
Eb.648	56
Eb.654	3
Eb.657	3
Eb.663	37, 38
Eb.669	40
Eb.689	3
Eb.722	27
Eb.732	3
Eb.733	37, 45
Eb.734	27
Eb.738	45, 55
Eb.741	33
Eb.749	33
Eb.751	3
Eb.755	55
Eb.756	24
Eb.762	38
Eb.770	40
Eb.776	28, 40
Eb.780	3
Eb.782	37, 40, 45
Eb.783	67
Eb.788	70
Eb.793	46
Eb.795	11, 24, 38, 46, 74
Eb.796	70
Eb.808	44, 46
Eb.813	27
Eb.845	37
Eb.847	37
Eb.854	24, 25, 27, 30, 31, 35, 40, 43, 70
Eb.855	25, 27, 31, 32, 33, 35
Eb.856	3, 31, 32, 33, 54, 70
Eb.857	26, 27, 33, 36, 43, 59
Eb.858	26, 33
Eb.859	33
Eb.862	33
Eb.867	26
Eb.869	33
Eb.871	33
Eb.873	27
Eb.874	26
Eb.877	26, 27

Edwin Smith Papyrus

Sm.1	24, 25, 30, 36, 40, 71
Sm.3	36
Sm.4	26, 36
Sm.5	36
Sm.6	25
Sm.7	25, 26
Sm.8	26, 34
Sm.9	37
Sm.11	42
Sm.12	34
Sm.18	25
Sm.19	25, 26
Sm.20	25
Sm.21	25, 26
Sm.22	25
Sm.25	42, 52
Sm.31	35
Sm.35	42
Sm.39	26
Sm.40	26
Sm.41	37
Sm.45	26
Sm.46	37, 39
Sm.48	25

Hearst Papyrus

He.53	55
He.55	55
He.56	55
He.59	37

www.ingramcontent.com/pod-product-compliance
Lightning Source LLC
Chambersburg PA
CBHW061007030426
42334CB00033B/3389